A12. 117770I £10-95

CW00515218

INTERPERSONAL SKILLS IN NURSING:
RESEARCH AND APPLICATIONS

Interpersonal Skills in Nursing
Research and Applications

Edited by Carolyn Kagan

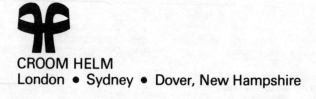

CROOM HELM
London • Sydney • Dover, New Hampshire

© 1985 Carolyn Kagan
Croom Helm Ltd, Provident House, Burrell Row, Beckenham, Kent BR3 1AT

Croom Helm Australia Pty Ltd, First Floor,
139 King Street, Sydney, NSW 2001, Australia

British Library Cataloguing in Publication Data
Interpersonal skills in nursing : research and applications
  1. Nurse and patient
  I. Kagan, Carolyn
610.73'06'99   RT86

ISBN 0-7099-1552-7

Croom Helm, 51 Washington Street, Dover, New Hampshire 03820, USA

Library of Congress Cataloging in Publication Data
Main entry under title:
Interpersonal Skills in Nursing
  Based on two conferences held at Manchester Polytechnic in 1982/83.
  Includes Index.
  1. Nurse and Patient — Congresses. 2. Interpersonal Relations — Congresses.
  I. Kagan, Carolyn. (DNLM: 1. Interpersonal Relations — Congresses.
  2. Nurses — Psychology — Congresses. WY 87 I613 1982-83)
RT86.3.I58   1985   610.73   85-9627
ISBN 0-7099-1552-7

Printed and bound in Great Britain
by Billing & Sons Limited, Worcester.

CONTENTS

*For
My Parents,
and
Amy and Anna*

PREFACE

This book is about interpersonal skills in nursing. It developed out of two conferences held at Manchester Polytechnic in 1982-3, on 'Interpersonal Skills in Nursing', and 'Teaching Interpersonal Skills in Nursing'. Each conference was well attended by practising nurses, nurse educators and psychologists who work with nurses in clinical and educational settings. The interest ranged from a quest for research information to a desire to exchange ideas about the implementation of research findings in nurse practice and education. I hope this book reflects these diverse interests.

In order to make some sense of what is written in this book, it is necessary to look and see who is writing it. Most of the authors will be familiar to nurses and/or psychologists, since they have spoken and written about their topics quite extensively. The contributions from nurses outnumber those from others (psychologists and psychiatrist) by ten to six, which is, I think, a reasonable balance. However, the men contributing outnumber the women by nine to six, which I do not think is a reasonable balance, but it is one that reflects the publishing status of men and women in psychology, and increasingly in nursing. In the field of interpersonal skills, arguably the most influential 'parent discipline' is psychology, itself a field that is dominated by male researchers asking male-defined questions: those women who struggle through the system to reach a position to research and/or publish, have been trained in this masculine field, and themselves ask similar questions and address similar issues. Nurses, too, who have backgrounds in the behavioural sciences, or who use the behavioural sciences to inform their work are also propagating these academic biases. The inquisitive reader should ask,

Would the questions asked and issues raised be different if more women were actively, involved in making their voices heard?

Carol Gillingham (1982) presents a convincing argument that they would.

A further observation about the contributors to this volume is that all except two of the nurses hold posts that involve nurse education in some form. I do not believe that this is because nurses in other fields do not have anything of importance or value to say: it is more likely to be an indication that clinical nurses have little time to devote to writing. Certainly, three clinical nurses who were invited to contribute to this book were unable to do so through lack of time, whereas only one 'nurse educator' withdrew for similar reasons. Again, the reader should ask,

Would the questions asked and the issues raised be different if more practising and clinical nurses were actively involved in making their voices heard?

In assessing the contents of this book, it is as important to speculate on what may have been excluded as to read what is included.

I do, however, apologise most sincerely to all those who have something to say, but who have not been given the opportunity, here, to say it: particularly to all those practising nurses, especially women, who simply do not have the time.

The book could not have proceeded without the interest and encouragement of Tim Hardwick of Croom Helm, and I would like to express my thanks to him. I am grateful to all the contributors for their commitment to their writing, their patience and tolerance of my handling of their works, and their understanding of my role as editor. I am indebted to my colleagues in the Nursing Section of the Polytechnic for their appreciative support of my Interpersonal Skills contributions to the various nursing courses; in particular, I owe a lot to the insightful and stimulating discussions I have had with Tony Butterworth and Brian Hodges.

I would like to express my gratitude to all the nursing students I have worked with over the years. The zeal with which they have participated in the (strangely) experiential interpersonal skills courses, and the readiness with which they have given me constructive criticism has maintained my spirits through periods of doubt. The enjoyment I get from my involvement with the subject is due, largely to them. My special thanks go to Eileen Barber, Sue Beales, Ernita Bhebhe, Katy Booth, Jo Bowers, Josie Evans, Barbara Fox, Janice Grant, Ennis Green, Shirley Hansell, Christine Howard, Lorraine Inglestone, Betty Kay, Angela Macfarlane, Debbie Major, Sue Mitchinson, Rosa Nicholson, John Rees, Rosie Smith, Steve Western and Eileen Yearn.

Several people have helped me prepare the book in different ways. Mrs Meehan and the women in the typing unit in the Faculty of Community Studies at the Polytechnic have dealt most efficiently with drafts of chapters presented to them in various states of disarray. I could not have spent so much time on the book without the help of Helen Burrows. Her creative and energetic work with my children has enabled me to combine teaching and writing with toddlers — and to survive! The person to whom I owe the most is Mark Burton. As well as writing a chapter himself, his belief that women should and must be heard has led him to postpone some of his own writing activities. Instead, he has undertaken more than his usual share of domestic chores, but is, I am sure, feminist enough to accept my thanks for the kind of help and support that women are generally expected to give to men.

Reference

Gillingham, C. (1982) *In A Different Voice: Psychological Theory and Women's Development*, Harvard University Press: Cambridge, Mass.

CONTRIBUTORS

Pat Ashworth, MSc, SRN, SCM, FRCN, Department of Nursing and Health Visiting, University of Ulster at Coleraine, Northern Ireland

Peter Banister, BA, PhD, ABPsS, Head of School of Psychology, Manchester Polytechnic, UK

Mark Burton, Senior Psychologist, Community Support Team for People with Mental Handicap, North Manchester Health Authority, UK

Desmond Cormack, PhD, Dip Ed, M Phil, Dip Nurs, RGN, RMN, Reader in Nursing, Department of Molecular and Life Sciences, Dundee College of Technology, UK

Colin Davidson, BA, MSc, Senior Lecturer in Psychology, School of Humanities and Contemporary Studies, Leeds Polytechnic *and* Honorary Clinical Psychologist, Leeds Area Health Authority (Western District), UK

Bryn D. Davis PhD, BSc, SRN, RMN, RNT, Principal Lecturer, Department of Community Studies, Brighton Polytechnic, UK

Ann Faulkner, MA, MLitt, SRN, RCNT, Dip Ed, Project Director CINE (Communication in Nurse Education), Department of Nursing, University of Manchester, UK

Carolyn Kagan, BSc, DPhil, Lecturer in Psychology (Social Psychology and Counselling), School of Psychology, Manchester Polytechnic, UK

Francis J. Lillie, District Psychologist, North East Essex and Mid-Essex Health Authorities, Colchester, UK

Jill Macleod Clark, PhD, BSc, SRN, Lecturer, Department of Nursing Studies, Chelsea College, University of London, UK

G. Peter Maguire, Senior Lecturer in Psychiatry, Department of Psychiatry, The University Hospital of South Manchester, UK

Gary Marshfield, BEd, SRN, RMN, RCNT, RNT, Nurse Tutor, Brighton School of Nursing, UK

Bill Reynolds, RMN, RGN, RNT, Nurse Teacher (Psychiatric Nursing), The Highland College of Nursing and Midwifery, Inverness, UK

Ann Tait, SRN, Dip. Adv. Soc. Studs., Vice-Chairman RCN Breast Care Nursing Forum (formerly Breast Care Specialist Nurse, Withington Hospital, Manchester, UK)

Anne Tomlinson, MSc, SRN, DipN (Lond.), RNT, Project Officer CINE (Communication in Nurse Education: An HEC Curriculum Development Project), Department of Nursing Studies, Chelsea College, University of London, UK

INTRODUCTION
Carolyn Kagan

Interpersonal Skills (IPS) are those aspects of both communication and social skills that are concerned with *direct person-to-person contact*. Communication (rightly) involves the passage of a message from sender to receiver through any medium, not only the interpersonal one. So, televised, tape-recorded and written messages are all forms of communication that may or may not be *interpersonal*. In the health field, social skills refer to many different facets of dealing with everyday life, not only the interpersonal ones. So, knowing how to dress, where to shop, how to use public transport and where to find a telephone number are all social skills that may or may not include *interpersonal* skills. We are, then, confining ourselves in this book to discussions of interpersonal aspects of communication and social skills in nursing. (For some discussions of the wider issues, see French, 1983; Smith and Bass, 1982. For examples of work where 'communication' refers to the interpersonal aspects of communication, see Bridge and Macleod Clark, 1981; Faulkner, 1984.)

It is worth, just for a moment, considering the assumptions behind a *skills* approach to social behaviour, as characterised by interest in social skills. In the UK, social skills training grew out of a model of social interaction (Argyle, 1967, 1969), stimulated by a growth in ergonomics (person-machine interaction). Argyle suggested that person-person interaction resembled person-machine interaction and could, similarly be broken down into 'stages' as indicated in Figure 1.1. Argyle and Kendon (1967) liken social skills to motor skills: both are conceptualised in terms of an integration of behaviours at a variety of different levels to produce smooth and co-ordinated responses to situations. Welford (1979) gives a stimulating historical account of a social skills approach to interaction in this country. Interest in the general approach has extended to focus on interaction 'problems', be they of psychologically disabled people (Trower, Bryant and Argyle, 1978), teachers (Flanders, 1970), managers (Sidney, Brown and Argyle, 1973), delinquent children and adolescents (Spence, 1982) or various professional groups (Ellis and Whittington, 1981), including nurses. For each of these groups, 'training' programmes have been devised, implemented and frequently evaluated. In recent years, many important conceptual and methodological issues have been raised that throw

Figure 1.1: A Model of Skilled Social Behaviour

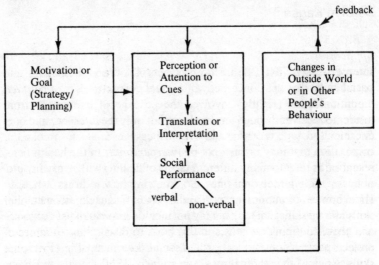

Source: Adapted from Argyle (1969)

doubt upon the optimism that has prevailed in a rapidly developing field (Ellis and Whittington, 1983; Spence and Shepherd, 1983; Trower, 1984).

There is a growing research literature relating to interpersonal skills in nursing and this is critically reviewed by several of the authors in this volume. As always, in the human relations field, the validity of research findings depends on more than the methods of particular studies. The discerning reader must ask 'Was the question the right one? 'Did the methods do justice to the people involved?' and the discerning practitioner must ask of the findings 'Does it happen like that?' 'Is this what my experience tells me? Throughout this collection, the (often uneasy) partnerships of research and application; theory and practice; and investigation and anecdote are revealed. Readers who find little in the research findings with which they can identify might more easily absorb the personal accounts: those who are frustrated by anecdote might discover insight from the research studies. Those who believe that nursing practice will only be advanced through knowledge accumulated by rigorous research practices will be relieved to find that the personal accounts included here are not subjectively biased and prejudiced accounts that leave themselves open to refutation. Instead, they are careful, genuine attempts to share experiences with readers, and as such they reflect a theme that is fundamental to an interpersonal skills approach to nursing — namely an open, non-defensive perspective on self, colleagues and patients.

Broadly, the book is organised along the dimension of '*research . . . applications*'. Part I provides the theoretical base for research into interpersonal skills in nursing. It includes a historical review of research paradigms, a discussion of research in (arguably) the most relevant parent field, and a critique of current research practices, pointing to future needs. Nursing cannot adopt the findings from other disciplines uncritically, owing to the context of nursing activities. In Part II, the context of nursing is examined from three different perspectives, representing the organisational, environmental and wider social contexts of nursing. Given the particular nature of the nursing profession, Part III examines the strengths and weaknesses of nurses' interpersonal skills and the effects these have on patient care in terms of psychosocial and physical recovery. This section, too, provides some examples of projects that have encouraged the more effective use of interpersonal skills. Arising out of these discussions is the issue of response to patient needs. The two chapters in Part IV consider interpersonal skills in relation to patients with greatly differing needs, referring to intensive care and mastectomy nursing.

Perhaps the single, most persistent plea to emerge from the research and accounts presented in the first four sections, is for more teaching/ training and learning in interpersonal skills to be developed. Part V deals exclusively with issues relating to the teaching and learning of interpersonal skills for nurses. Methods of teaching and learning, schemes for teaching different groups of nurses in training and the central question of evaluation are all addressed.

Finally, the *Postscript* allows me to draw out and reflect upon some of the themes, and to consider the implications for future research and application. The book will have succeeded if it stimulates you to do the same.

References

Argyle, M. (1967) *The Psychology of Interpersonal Behaviour*, Penguin: Harmondsworth (1st edition)
Argyle, M. (1969) *Social Interaction*, Methuen: London

Argyle, M. and Kendon, A. (1967) 'The Experimental Analysis of Social Performance' in L. Berkowitz (ed.), *Advances in Experimental Social Psychology*, *3*, Academic Press: New York

Bridge, W. and Macleod Clark, J. (eds) (1981) *Communication in Nursing Care*, HM & M: Aylesbury

Ellis, R.A.F. and Whittington, D. (1981) *A Guide to Social Skill Training*, Croom Helm: London

Ellis, R.A.F. and Whittington, D. (eds) (1983) *New Directions in Social Skills Training*, Croom Helm: London

Faulkner, A. (ed.) (1984) *Recent Advances in Nursing*, *7*, *Communication* Churchill Livingstone, Edinburgh

Flanders, N.A. (1970) *Analyzing Teaching Behavior*, Addison Wesley: Reading, Mass.

French, P. (1983) *Social Skills for Nursing Practice*, Croom Helm: London

Sidney, E., Brown, M. and Argyle, M. (1973) *Skills with People: A Guide for Managers*, Hutchinson: London

Smith, V.M. and Bass, T.A. (1982) *Communication for the Health Care Team* (adapted by A. Faulkner) Harper and Row: London

Spence, S. (1982) *Social Skills Training with Children and Adolescents*, NFER: Windsor, Berks.

Spence, S. and Shepherd, G. (1983) *Developments in Social Skills Training*, Academic Press: London

Trower, P. (ed.) (1984) *Radical Approaches to Social Skills Training*, Croom Helm: London

Trower, P., Bryant, B. and Argyle, M. (1978) *Social Skills and Mental Health*, Methuen: London

Welford, A.T. (1979) 'The Concept of Skill and its Application to Social Performance' in W.T. Singleton, P. Spurgeon and R.B. Stammers (eds) *The Analysis of Social Skill*, Plenum: New York

PART I:

THE THEORETICAL BACKGROUND TO INTERPERSONAL SKILLS IN NURSING

EDITORIAL INTRODUCTION

Interest in the area of interpersonal skills in nursing has been evident for many years, as *Jill Macleod Clark* shows in her historical review of research studies, in *Chapter 1*. The methods of research have changed over the years, increasing in sophistication from surveys of patient satisfaction to interaction and observation studies. Whilst the findings of many of these studies have been considered by Government bodies or committees for some time, it is only recently that nursing authorities have firmly incorporated specific interpersonal skills issues into policy (and training) statements. This recognition has led to a number of curriculum development studies and attempts to evaluate the impact of different teaching methods. Macleod Clark suggests that more research of this type is needed if interpersonal skills training is to develop usefully.

Whilst all the research paradigms reviewed are still currently in use, the changes in research methods here have paralleled developments in other fields, especially the social sciences, which have, for a long time studied matters of relevance to the interpersonal aspects of interaction. Various theoretical antecedents in the parent disciplines have given rise to many of the issues of current concern to nurses. In *Chapter 2*, *Colin Davidson* examines the lessons to be learnt from work in both assertion training and social skills training. Davidson offers a comprehensive, selective review of the numerous studies into the nature of skilled social behaviour and the effectiveness of training, stemming from the social/clinical psychology field. The work in social skills training has pointed to the role of cognitive factors in both interpersonal skill and effective training, the need to consider different levels of skills and subskills when examining complex social behaviour, and the need to determine which components of a training package are the effective ones. Davidson draws attention to some of the critiques of the liberal and often indiscriminate use of social skills training that have emerged, and that nurses would be well advised to heed.

He points out the problems that have been found with the assessment of skilled social behaviour and the evaluation of training, and attempts to encourage the generalisation of skills across different settings. Skilled behaviour is, he notes, a complex interaction of emotional factors (such as anxiety), skill factors (such as displaying the appropriate

7

verbal and non-verbal behaviours, and accurately perceiving social events), and cognitive factors (such as beliefs about oneself and one's own social competence). Any consideration of interpersonal skills in nursing should take all these factors into account. Another lesson to be drawn from the literature on social skills training relates to the importance of 'interaction partners' for determining the acceptability of particular skilled behaviours, as opposed to the 'expert' researchers or trainers.

The question of who decides which interpersonal skills are appropriate, and when acceptable levels of skill have been reached, is picked up by *Peter Banister and Carolyn Kagan* in *Chapter 3*. They examine the wisdom of drawing extensively on the literature from other fields, and suggest that this might be inappropriate, as the nurse-patient relationship is a special one. The pressures that are brought to bear on nurses and patients to adhere to their roles, and the attendant expectations held by everyone around them define their relationship as special. Furthermore, attention is drawn to the importance of doctors in defining the interaction context of much of nursing. They argue, too, that the process of borrowing research findings and paradigms from other disciplines frequently ignores the very theoretical debates and critiques that have emerged. This, they suggest, has happened in the field of interpersonal skills in nursing: many theoretical issues in, for example, social psychology, have not been incorporated into the planning, execution and interpretation of research data. For the future, Banister and Kagan urge that first, the prevailing (empiricist) traditions of research in this area be challenged, so that a more humanistic view of participants in the research is taken; second, that the meaning of the interpersonal behaviours for all concerned be accounted for; and third, that whole interaction context be examined and note taken of the special features of the context(s) in which nursing takes place.

1 THE DEVELOPMENT OF RESEARCH IN INTERPERSONAL SKILLS IN NURSING

Jill Macleod Clark

Introduction

Social scientists and nurses have been exploring the area of communication and interpersonal skills in nursing for at least two decades, using a variety of methods and approaches. For a long time these studies made little apparent impact on professional practice. More recently there has been a growing recognition of the central role of communication in nursing practice and the need for interpersonal skills training in nursing and training.

This chapter charts the development of communication research in nursing, emphasising points where the research has had some effect on practice and policy and highlighting areas where more research is needed.

Historical Development

It is interesting to speculate why it has taken so long for the importance of communication and interpersonal skills in nursing to be recognised. It could and should have happened decades ago. Table 1.1 shows in a simplistic way the overall development of research approaches in this area in the UK.

Table 1.1: Development of U.K. Research in Communication and Interpersonal Skills in Nursing

Patient satisfaction surveys	(1960s — present)
Intervention and quasi-experimental studies demonstrating benefits of improved communication	(1970s — present)
Observation studies, describing and analysing nurse-patient interaction	(1970s — present)
Studies of the effectiveness of interpersonal skills teaching	(1980s — present)

9

The earliest studies were surveys of patients' satisfaction with the care they received (McGhee, 1961). The next main group of studies were those that fall into the quasi-experimental paradigm where an attempt is made to measure the benefits of increased or improved communication between nurses and patients. There is generally an intervention in the form of giving patients specific information (e.g. Boore, 1978; Hayward, 1975). This kind of research continued, as did the surveys, while alongside it developed the descriptive, observation studies of interaction between nurses and patients in a variety of settings (e.g. Bond, 1981; Wells, 1975). As time went on the methods used by researchers became more sophisticated and analysis tended to become more detailed. The most recent research developments in interpersonal skills in nursing have tended to move from the analysis of nurse-patient interaction, into the classroom. Recognition of the need to teach interpersonal skills to nurses has led to a number of curriculum development studies (e.g. Faulkner, Macleod Clark and Bridge, 1983). Attempts are also being made to evaluate the effectiveness of using different methods to teach interpersonal skills (e.g. Ellis, 1980).

All the types of research listed above will be discussed in more detail in the following sections of this chapter. However, it is important to bear in mind that the chronological development is only approximate and there is much overlap between types of study in historical terms.

Surveys of Patient Satisfaction

Over the past two decades many researchers have investigated, either directly or indirectly, the extent to which patients are satisfied with the care they receive. In general it has been shown that patients are satisfied neither with communication in general nor the amount of information they receive. A common thread between these studies is the finding that patients are frequently more critical about poor communication between staff and patients than about any other aspect of their experience in hospital. For example, McGhee (1961) used an unstructured questionnaire to interview 490 patients within two weeks of their discharge from surgical and medical wards of a Scottish hospital. McGhee found that each patient referred to aspects of communication and 65 per cent of them were actually dissatisfied with this part of their care. In this study communication was the single largest source of dissatisfaction with, by comparison, approximately 40 per cent of the sample complaining about 'noise' and approximately 30 per cent being dissatisfied with aspects of their medical care.

In 1964, Cartwright used a structured interview schedule to interview 739 people who had been in hospital during the previous six months. The schedule covered many aspects of the patients' experiences during and after hospitalisation. The outstanding finding of this survey was that 29 per cent of all patients in the sample expressed serious dissatisfaction with communication, while 61 per cent mentioned some degree of dissatisfaction with communication. Patients were also asked how much information their ward sister had given them about their illness, treatment or progress. 16 per cent said 'a lot', 40 per cent said 'a little' and 44 per cent said 'none'. The remainder of the nursing staff were found to have given very little information to the patients.

Hugh-Jones, Tanser and Whitby (1964) explored the anxieties and dissatisfaction of a sample of 245 medical ward patients. They found that even though the staff involved had made an effort to explain diagnosis and treatment, 39 per cent were dissatisfied with the amount of information they received. It is frequently suggested that patients' recall is poor (Bradshaw, Ley and Kinsey 1975; Ley and Spelman, 1967) and that dissatisfaction is due to this factor. However, Hugh-Jones *et al.* found that recall of information actually given to patients was accurate in 79 per cent of the patients. This finding of dissatisfaction with the amount of information given was confirmed by Raphael (1969), and in a review of studies of patient satisfaction Ley (1972) concluded that many patients are not satisfied with the amount and/or type of information given to them in hospital. Skeet (1970) investigated the needs of patients recently discharged from hospital and also found that many patients, particularly the elderly, were discharged without having been given adequate information, preparation, instruction or advice. Eardley, Davis and Wakefield (1975) found that patients who were expected to cope with chronic disability were given inadequate explanation, education and advice. More recently, in a study of surgical patients, Reynolds (1978) asked 100 patients specifically about the information they had received about their illness and treatment, and found that over 50 per cent were dissatisfied with the information given.

The findings of many of the research studies discussed above have, over the years, been noted by various government bodies or committees. Recommendations for improvement in staff-patient communication have been made in a variety of documents (CHSC, 1963; CNO, 1977; DHSS, 1976), but the fact remains that patients' complaints about poor communication have continued to rise. For example, in

1978 the NHS Ombudsman reported:

> During the year I issued 120 reports of investigations into individual
> complaints . . . There is one underlying consideration which seems
> to me to be present in most, if not all cases. This is the problem of
> communication . . .
>
> (HMSO, 1978).

Most importantly, an increasing proportion of these complaints were
found to be directed towards nursing staff (DHSS, 1973; HMSO,
1979). Thus it can be seen that the results of the studies reviewed above
could, in theory, have resulted in direct action in terms of improving
nurse-patient communication. Initially, however, the reality proved to
be somewhat different with the emphasis in research concentrating on
quasi-experimental studies such as those described below.

Intervention Studies

Most intervention studies follow a similar experimental design involving a large group of patients who have similar medical treatment. From
this main group, patients are then randomly allocated to either the
experimental group or the control group. The patients in the experimental group receive additional information from and interaction with the
researcher while patients allocated to the control group receive routine
treatment but receive no additional information, although they may get
additional attention from the researcher in terms of interaction time. All
patients in these studies are then compared in terms of physiological or
psychological measures.

Most of the early studies of this type were undertaken by researchers in
the USA. Egbert *et al.* (1964) found that anaesthetists giving patients
pre-operative instructions and encouragement significantly reduced
post-operative pain. In a series of studies, Johnson (Johnson, 1965/6;
Johnson, Morrissey and Leventhal, 1973) analysed the effect of purposeful nurse-patient interaction, designed to enable patients to gain
accurate expectations of discomfort, on post-operative condition and
behaviour. She also analysed the contribution of emotional response
processes in adaptation to surgery (Johnson, 1971). These studies have
demonstrated that giving patients *realistic* expectations of their post-
operative state can significantly reduce the levels of anxiety and stress
experienced. Johnson, Kirchhoff and Endress (1975) have also examined
the effect of giving children a more accurate picture of what is going to

happen to them during plaster cast removal, and have shown that children with realistic expectations have less pain and are less distressed during the procedure.

More recently, similar studies were carried out in the UK. For example, Hayward (1975) found that patients in the experimental group, given specific pre-operative information, required significantly fewer analgesic drugs than patients in the control group. This finding was substantiated by Boore (1978), who showed that giving surgical patients pre-operative information resulted in a reduction in post-operative 'stress' as determined by physiological measures. In Boore's study the dependent variables were excretion of 17-hydroxycorticosteroids, sodium and potassium in urine, body temperatures and post-operative complications, in addition to the amount of pain experienced and analgesics administered.

Other studies have examined the effect of giving carefully prepared explanations to patients undergoing investigations such as gastroscopy (Johnson *et al*, 1973) and barium meal or barium enema (Wilson-Barnett, 1978). In the study by Johnson it was found that patients who did not receive the explanation required significantly more sedation than the groups of patients who did. Moreover, the group which received realistic information related to the sensations they would experience, also had significantly lower tension scores than both the control group and the group who received factual information only. Wilson-Barnett found that patients given an explanation before barium enema reported significantly less anxiety than patients who had not received the explanation. Interestingly, however, no significant differences were found amongst patients undergoing barium meal investigations, in terms of the effect of explanation on anxiety levels. (Chapter 9 by Bryn Davis explores this issue further.)

All the studies described above have important implications in terms of the relevance of some aspects of communication to effective nursing care. Overall, they demonstrate the value of increased interaction and of giving information and explanation to patients undergoing stressful operations, procedures or events, in terms of reducing pain, anxiety, vomiting and other side effects. Clearly such studies have important implications for nursing practice in terms of the nurse's contribution to the task of informing or reassuring patients about treatment. However, they should also be examined critically on a number of counts. Firstly, these studies show what happened when the *researcher* (admittedly, often a nurse) gave patients additional time or information. Thus the research quoted only demonstrates the effectiveness of 'outside' or additional individuals as communicators. To date, little research has been undertaken to evaluate the effect on patients of the actual ward staff giving additional information. One study (Davis, 1981) has examined this problem, and found it necessary to teach the nurses concerned 'communication skills' in order to enable them to inform and explain to patients in an appropriate way.

The second question which needs to be asked of these experimental research studies concerns individual differences. There is an implicit assumption underlying these studies that all patients benefit from additional information and indeed that they all benefit from the *same* information. The findings of Wilson-Barnett (1978) cast some doubt on this assumption. She found that the effect of giving information varied according to the investigation being undergone and that there were large individual variations in response to receiving information. Andrew (1967) also found that surgical patients' personality traits influenced the effect that pre-operative information had on their post-operative recovery period. Therefore, although as a generalisation patients appear to benefit from additional information, the response of individual patients can vary enormously. There is clearly a need for further studies to explore differences in patients' needs for information and support — differences which may be related to variables such as the patient's age, sex, diagnosis, education, culture and so on.

Perhaps the most vital question related to these experimental studies is concerned with the differences between nurses in terms of their skills as informants and communicators. This is a problem which has had to be faced in field studies in which the effect of giving information to patients is investigated (Davis, 1981), and where early findings suggest that nurses possess limited communication skills. Such findings are not surprising given the results of the studies reviewed in the next section, namely the description and analysis of nurse-patient interaction.

Observation Studies

An essential prerequisite of nurse-patient communication is nurse-patient contact, and the very earliest studies in this area were, in fact, 'time and motion' studies. The motivation for this research was often related to the need to analyse nurses' work in order to establish methods of allocating staff and resources. The analysis of nurses' work in these studies tended to illustrate that relatively little time was spent in one-to-one conversation or communication with patients. For example, Oppenheim (1955) found that 'talking with patients' took less than 10 per cent of the nurses' time on psychiatric wards.

Over a period of time researchers have moved towards a more specific study of nurse-patient interaction in a variety of different clinical settings. It is possible to trace a pattern of increasingly detailed analysis and increasingly sophisticated data collection methods over the past ten or fifteen years. Studies in psychiatric nursing by Altschul, (1972) and Cormack (1976) described the overall pattern and structure of nurse-patient interactions. This research highlighted the limitations in both quantity and quality of communication. More recent work by Macilwaine (1980) focused on a specific group of psychiatric patients (neurotics) and attempted a detailed analysis of nurse-patient conversations in this area using tape-recorded data. Macilwaine also found a picture of superficial interactions which were limited in quality and quantity, and were predominantly related to nursing tasks or administration. There was little evidence of nurses giving emotional support or developing therapeutic relationships with these patients.

Studies which have examined interaction between nurses and geriatric patients have produced similarly depressing findings, with nurses spending only 1 to 4 per cent of their time in conversation with patients (Adams and McIlwraith, 1963; Norton, McLaren and Exton-Smith, 1976; Stockwell, 1972). A more recent study in this area by Wells (1975), again showed that approximately 4 per cent of nurses' time was spent in personal contact with patients although there were large individual nurse and ward differences. By using tape recordings, Wells was able to measure the length of interactions with accuracy and confirmed previous findings of short exchanges between nurses and geriatric patients. More than half of the exchanges recorded lasted for less than 25 seconds, and the average length of interactions was 1 minute 28 seconds.

This trend towards the use of more sophisticated recording techniques and detailed analysis of interaction is most marked in studies of nurses and patients on general medical and surgical wards. Earlier studies, such as those by Dodd (1974) and Franklin (1974), identified the limitations of nurse-patient interactions in a general way. Much more specific information about such interactions is now available in relation to nurses and surgical patients (Macleod Clark, 1981, 1982) and nurses and medical patients (Faulkner, 1980). Faulkner attempted to describe the student nurses' role in giving information to patients, and used a radio-microphone to tape-record conversations between nurses and patients. These recordings were then selectively transcribed and coded in terms of the information giving or receiving which took place. She found that the average length of interactions was between 2 and 3 minutes and that many of the patients' questions were left unanswered. The study of communication between nurses and patients on surgical wards undertaken by Macleod Clark (1981, 1982) took both the recording and the analysis processes a stage further. Recordings were made using radio-microphone equipment and videotape equipment, and a random sample of all recorded conversations was analysed in great depth, using a variety of coding strategies. The results from this study again confirmed quantitative limitations in nurse-patient conversations, with a median conversation length of 1.13 minutes, and with nurses spending less than 14 per cent of time in contact with patients. Conversational topics were superficial and task related and the majority were initiated by the nurses.

The conversations were also analysed in terms of the interpersonal skills required to initiate and maintain conversation such as questioning, attending, reinforcing and responding. Results of this analysis revealed that the nurses in the study demonstrated little evidence of interpersonal skills. Their questions to patients were nearly always closed or leading, with few examples of open questioning. Reinforcing or encouraging strategies were rarely used appropriately and there was evidence of a lack of listening and attending. Nurses' responses to patients' questions and cues were often negative in that over half the responses or answers were evasive, clichéd or even absent. The overall picture was one of tactics that discouraged communication rather than skills that encouraged it.

Evidence from research such as that of Macleod Clark (1982) described above, has lent weight to the arguments currently being put forward for the need to incorporate the teaching of interpersonal skills into programmes of nurse education. Until recently, this aspect of teaching has been neglected in the UK. While the subject is sometimes taught during psychiatric nurse training (Dietrich, 1978), interpersonal or communication skills have neither been taught nor formally assessed in courses leading to general nurse training (Faulkner *et al.*, 1983; Nurse, 1977) or in post-basic courses (Bridge and Speight, 1981). In the USA however, communication skills teaching is specifically included in most training programmes (Ceriale, 1976; Sparks *et al.*, 1980). Introducing interpersonal or communication skills into a curriculum will have implications in terms of time and resources, and it is important to be able to assess the feasibility and outcome of such changes. Indeed, Gary Marshfield, Carolyn Kagan and Bill Reynolds, in Part V, discuss some of these implications in the context of different training courses. In the next section, research which has attempted to examine the impact and effectiveness of teaching interpersonal skills in nursing and related professions is reviewed.

Studies of the Impact and Effectiveness of Teaching Interpersonal Skills

There are a number of different approaches commonly used in interpersonal skill training, and these approaches in turn use a variety of teaching methods. As a general rule, methods are experiential; that is, the student has to participate in the learning process and experience learning through feelings as well as increased knowledge and insight. (See Anne Tomlinson's review of experiential teaching/learning methods in Chapter 12.)

These methods are not easy to assess objectively, many requiring the students themselves to determine the extent of learning on a subjective basis. For example, many exercises are used in communication skills teaching specifically to help the student increase his or her level of self-awareness. Assessing the effectiveness of such teaching must inevitably be based upon the students' subjective perceptions of their own self-awareness. Jasmin and Hill (1978) found that video-taped self-image confrontation was a powerful means of developing insight and self-awareness. Fielding (1983) also demonstrated that video-taped stimulus material increased students' awareness of the importance of communication. People do vary, though, in their reactions to video-taped self-confrontation: just as some develop insight, others become self-conscious and very anxious (Buss, 1980).

Many teachers in this field feel that empathy is an important skill, or set of skills, for students to develop. The literature describing attempts to teach and assess empathy levels is large and diverse, spanning many groups of health professionals including social workers, doctors and counsellors. In the USA studies have been undertaken to monitor the effect of empathy training on groups of nurses. The training usually consists of a theoretical introduction followed by the modelling and role-playing practice. Increase in empathic skill is measured using a scale such as the Carkhuff scale (Carkhuff, 1971). Kalisch (1971) found that nurses only registered small increases on the scale scoring an average of 1.5 on a 5 point scale. La Monica (1976) found similar results and pointed out that baseline empathy scores in nurses tended to be very low, even after training. Carkhuff (1971) has suggested that in order to communicate sensitively with patients or clients, professionals should achieve an empathy score of at least 3.0. In La Monica's study only three out of thirty-nine nurses in the group achieved this score.

Many other communication teaching programmes are based on the principle of training students to use specific interpersonal skills appropriately. This approach is based on the original microteaching programmes for teachers during the 1960s (Allen and Ryan, 1969). These have been adapted by a number of teachers and researchers for the development of skills relevant to nurses and other health professionals. Teaching for skills training generally follows a pattern of skill analysis followed by practice, followed by individual feedback on performance for each student. (Colin Davidson gives a detailed account of this process in Chapter 2.) Students' performance can be assessed using rating scales or observation schedules, and comparisons can be made between groups of students who have undergone training and similar groups who have not.

Most studies of this kind consistently demonstrate improvements after training in students' performance on a variety of skills such as listening, questioning and reinforcing. Ellis (1980) describes performance increments in health visitors and social workers, and Ivey and Authier (1978) show improvements in counselling skills in a variety of health professionals. Although many of the studies of performance increment can be criticised on methodological grounds in terms of 'teaching the test', the results are encouraging. Subjective evaluations from students are also positive (Rackham and Morgan, 1977), and some methods of monitoring and recording personal progress are reviewed by Jones (1984) and by Bill Reynolds (Chapter 14). Such 'process recording' is interesting as it serves the dual purpose of training and evaluation.

Conclusion

The evidence demonstrating that nurses need to develop their communication skills is overwhelming and there are significant changes emerging in the design of nursing curricula as a consequence. Some attempts are currently being made to monitor the impact of inserting communication skills as a taught and assessed component in nurse education programmes (Neeson *et al.*, 1984). Such innovations have inevitable implications in terms of the skills and experience of the teachers responsible for nurse education.

More research is needed to examine the relative impact and effectiveness of different methods of teaching interpersonal skills to student nurses. There is some evidence that experiential learning methods such as role play and video feedback have to be introduced cautiously when dealing with young and inexperienced students (Tomlinson, Macleod Clark and Faulkner, 1984). In the meantime, while curriculum developments continue, further work is being undertaken on the observation and analysis of nurse-patient communication. Such studies are vital if an understanding of the complex dynamics of professional interaction is to develop.

References

Adams, G.F. and McIlwraith, P.L. (1963) *Geriatric Nursing*, Oxford University Press: London

Allen, D. and Ryan, K. (1969) *Microteaching*, Addison-Wesley: Reading, Mass.

Altschul, A. (1972) Patient-Nurse Interaction, Churchill Livingstone: Edinburgh

Andrew, J.M. (1967) 'Coping Styles, Stress Relevant Learning and Recovery from Surgery', unpublished PhD thesis: University of California

Bond, S. (1981) 'Communicating with Cancer Patients' in W. Bridge and J. Macleod Clark (eds), *Communication in Nursing Care*, HM and M (Wiley): Aylesbury, Bucks.

Boore, J. (1978) *A Prescription for Recovery*, Royal College of Nursing: London

Bradshaw, P., Ley, P. and Kinsey, J.A. (1975) 'Recall of Medical Advice', *British Journal of Social and Clinical Psychology*, *14*, 55-62

Bridge, W. and Speight, I. (1981) 'Teaching the Skills of Nursing Communication', *Nursing Times*, 77, 125-7

Buss, A.H. (1980) *Self Consciousness and Social Anxiety*, Freeman: San Francisco

Carkhuff, R. (1971) *The Development of Human Resources*, Holt, Rinehart and Winston: New York

Cartwright, A. (1964) *Human Relations and Hospital Care*, Routledge and Kegan Paul: London

Ceriale, L. (1976) 'Facilitated Unfolding of Human Relation Skills in the Baccalaureate Nursing Student', *Nursing Educator*, September/October, 11-14

CHSC (1963) *Communications Between Doctors, Nurses and Patients*, Central Health Services Council and Ministry of Health, HMSO: London

CNO (1977) *Communication with Patients*, Chief Nursing Officers Letter No. 14. Standards of Nursing Care, DHSS: London

Cormack, D. (1976) *Psychiatric Nursing Observed*, RCN: London

Davis, B. (1981) 'Pre-operative Information Giving in Relation to Patient Outcome', *Nursing Times*, 77, 599-601

DHSS (1973) *Report of Committee on Hospital Complaints Procedure*, HMSO: London

DHSS (1976) *The Organisation of the In-patient's Day, HMSO: London*

Dietrich, G. (1978) 'Teaching Psychiatric Nursing in the Classroom', *Journal of Advanced Nursing, 3*, 525-34

Dodd, A.P. (1974) 'Towards an Understanding of Nursing', unpublished PhD thesis: University of London

Eardley, A., Davis, F. and Wakefield, J. (1975) 'Health Education by Chance: The unmet need of patients in hospital and after', *International Journal of Health Education*, *18*, 1

Egbert, L., Battit, G., Welch, C. and Bartlett, M. (1964) 'Reduction of Post-operative Pain by Encouragement and Instruction of Patients', *New England Journal of Medicine*, *270*, 825-7

Ellis, R. (1980), 'Social Skills Training for the Interpersonal Professions' in W. Singleton, P. Spurgeon, and R. Stammers (eds), *The Analysis of Social Skill*, Plenum: New York

Faulkner, A. (1980) 'Communication and the Nurse', *Nursing Times*, *76*, 93-5

Faulkner, A., Macleod, Clark, J. and Bridge, W. (1983) *Teaching Communication in Schools of Nursing* Paper given at RCN Research Conference: Brighton

Fielding, P. (1983) 'An Evaluation of Videotaped Teaching Material', Unpublished report, King Edward's Hospital Fund for London: London

Franklin, P. (1974) *Patient Anxiety on Admission to Hospital*, Royal College of Nursing: London

Hayward, J. (1975) *Information — A Prescription Against Pain*, Royal College of Nursing: London

HMSO (1978) Health Services Commissioner — *Annual Report of Session 1977-1978*, HMSO: London

HMSO (1979) Health Services Commissioner — *Annual Report of Session 1978-1979*, HMSO: London

Hugh-Jones, P., Tanser, A. and Whitby, C. (1964) 'Patients' View of Admission to a London Teaching Hospital', *British Medical Journal*, *9*, 660-4

Ivey, A. and Authier, R. (1978) *Microcounselling*, C.C. Thomas: New York

Jasmin, S. and Hill, L. (1978) 'Videotaping and Interpersonal Skill Development', *Nursing Leadership*, *1*, 4-10

Johnson, J. (1965/66) 'Influence of Purposeful Nurse-patient Interaction on the Patient's Post-operative Course' in *Exploring Progress in Medical Surgical Nursing Practice*, American Nurses Association: New York

Johnson, J. (1971) 'Contribution of Emotional and Instrumental Response Processes in Adaptation to Surgery', *Journal of Personality and Social Psychology*, *20*, 55-64

Johnson, J., Kirchhoff, K. and Endress, M. (1975) 'Altering Children's Distress Behaviour During Orthopaedic Cast Removal', *Nursing Research*, *24*, 404-10

Johnson, J., Morrisey, J. and Leventhal, H. (1973) 'Psychological Preparation for Endoscopic Examination', *Gastrointestinal Endoscopy*, *19*, 180-2

Jones, C.M. (1984) 'Process Recording for Communication with Psychiatric Patients — Techniques for Improving Skills of Communication', in A. Faulkner (ed.) *Recent Advances in Nursing*, *7*, *Communication*, Churchill Livingstone: Edinburgh

Kalisch, B. (1971) 'Strategies for Developing Nurse Empathy', *Nursing Outlook*, *19*, 714-8

La Monica, E. (1976) 'Empathy Training', *Nursing Research*, *25*, 447-51

Ley, P. (1972) 'Complaints Made By Hospital Staff and Patients: A review of the literature', *Bulletin of British Psychological Society*, *25*, 115-20

Ley, P. and Spelman, M. (1967) *Communicating with the Patient*, Staples Press: London

Macilwaine, H. (1980) 'The Nursing of Female Neurotic Patients in Psychiatric Units of General Hospitals', unpublished PhD thesis: University of Manchester

Macleod Clark, J. (1981) 'Nurse-Patient Communication', *Nursing Times*, *77*, 12-18

Macleod Clark, J. (1982) *Nurse-Patient Interaction. An Analysis of Conversations on Surgical Wards*, Unpublished PhD Thesis: University of London

McGhee, A. (1961) *The Patients' Attitude to Nursing Care*, Churchill Livingstone: Edinburgh

Neeson, B., Bridge, W., Faulkner, A. and Macleod Clark, J. (1984) 'Teaching Communication Skills to Nurses': Parts 1 and 2, *Nurse Education Today, 4*, 2 and 3

Norton, D., McLaren, R. and Exton-Smith, A. (1976) *An Investigation of Geriatric Nursing Problems in Hospital* (Reprint) Churchill Livingstone: Edinburgh

Nurse, G. (1977) *The Professional Helping Relationship and its Relevance for Nurse Education*, Unpublished Dip Ed Thesis: Institute of Education, University of London

Oppenheim, A. (1955) *The Function and Training of Mental Nurses*, Chapman and Hall: London

Rackham, N. and Morgan, J. (1977) *Behaviour Analysis in Training*, McGraw Hill: Maidenhead

Raphael, W. (1969) *Patients and their Hospitals*, King Edward's Hospital Fund for London: London

Reynolds, M. (1978) 'No News is Bad News: Patients' views about communication in hospital', *British Medical Journal, 1*, 1673-76

Skeet, M. (1970) *Home from Hospital*, Dan Mason Nursing Research Committee: London

Sparks, S., Vitalo, P., Cohen, B. and Kahn, G. (1980) 'Teaching of Interpersonal Skills to Nurse Practitioner Students', *Journal of Continuing Education in Nursing, 11*, 5-16

Stockwell, F. (1972) *The Unpopular Patient*, Royal College of Nursing: London (Republished by Croom Helm, London, 1984)

Tomlinson, A., Macleod Clark, J. and Faulkner, A. (1984) 'The Use of Role Play in Nurse Education': Part 1, *Nursing Times, 80*, 38, 48-51; Part 2, *Nursing Times, 80*, 39, 45-47

Wells, T. (1975) *Problems in Geriatric Nursing Care*, Churchill Livingstone: Edinburgh

Wilson-Barnett, J. (1978) 'Patients' Emotional Responses to Barium X-rays', *Journal of Advanced Nursing, 3*, 37-46

2 THE THEORETICAL ANTECEDENTS TO INTERPERSONAL SKILLS TRAINING

Colin Davidson

Introduction

There are many theoretical antecedents to interpersonal skills training, emerging from fields as diverse as ergonomics, dynamic psychiatry, behavioural psychology, humanistic psychology, and, with the advent of the audio and then the video recorder, microteaching. However, for the purposes of this chapter I shall limit the discussion to those antecedents which focus on the idea that skilled interpersonal behaviour is analogous to other types of skill and all that that implies, particularly that:

(1) it is learnt, mislearnt or forgotten in much the same way as other behaviours;

(2) it can be broken down into component or constituent parts that can each be considered separately and combined to produce generalised skill;

(3) appropriate training for its development can be adequately devised, tested and evaluated.

I shall concentrate on these approaches for several reasons. Firstly, it is the framework that a number of professions have adopted in attempts to enhance the effectiveness of their members, particularly in the 'human service' professions such as teaching, medicine, management and nursing. (See, for example, Argyle, 1981a, b; Ellis and Whittington, 1981; Wilkinson and Canter, 1982, for illustrations in this country.) Secondly, it is the approach that many nurses will (have been trained to) use in encouraging interpersonal effectiveness in their clients. Thirdly, discussion of the theoretical antecedents of social skills training raises many pertinent issues for nursing, if it seeks to apply knowledge, methods and procedures from other disciplines.

22

This critical review of social skills training (SST) focuses on a number of issues that emerge from the literature:

(1) the identification of skills or components of skills which can be trained;

(2) the development of ways of conceptualising social behaviour within a 'skills' framework;

(3) a consideration of the importance of integrating cognitive factors with earlier formulations;

(4) the role of videotape recordings;

(5) the identification of the effective components in social skills training programmes;

(6) mutual assessments and assessment of progress and outcome;

(7) the short and long term effects of training and the problems of promoting generalisation of training;

(8) some wider social considerations raised by training programmes.

I have discussed work in SST with reference to applications of the training (techniques) to clients with psychological problems in order to illustrate and develop the above points.

In 1979 I participated with a group of psychiatric nurses in establishing a social skills training programme on a psychiatric unit (Davidson, 1980). It was a short step for most of the team to realise that the techniques we were planning to use with patients could be used equally effectively to develop our own skills as professional helpers. In the brief historical review that follows, I hope the reader will be able to make a similar shift, from the early psychiatric context of this approach to the wider issue of the development of the interpersonal skills of the professional helper. Before doing this, it may be useful to consider in more detail the foundations of SST in (a) assertion training, and (b) analysis of social interaction.

Assertion Training

Wolpe (1969) put forward the view that many patients have 'unadaptive anxiety responses that prevent them from saying or doing what is reasonable and right'. He argued that this inhibition and the suppression of feelings to which it gives rise may lead to prolonged states of arousal, which may in turn produce 'somatic symptoms and even pathological changes in predisposed organs'. Recent research into life events (Rahe *et al.*, 1974) supports Wolpe's view concerning the long term consequences of emotional stress. Wolpe devised a package of assertion training techniques (Wolpe and Lazarus, 1966) designed to enable patients to develop socially acceptable ways of expressing negative reactions to situations. This package consisted of a combination of counter-conditioning, behaviour rehearsal, modelling, instructions, coaching, feedback, social reinforcement and homework assignments.

The sorts of things that training focused on can be illustrated by an item from the Behavioral Assertiveness Test (Hersen, Eisler and Miller, 1973). The patient is told:

> You're in a crowded grocery store in a hurry. You pick one small item and get in line to pay for it. You're really trying to hurry because you're already late for an appointment. Then a woman with a shopping cart full of groceries cuts in line in front of you. She says 'You don't mind if I cut in here do you? I'm in a hurry'.

After being given this scene the patient is then asked to role-play her/his response with a female research assistant. Unassertive patients might be provided with videotaped models of other people dealing with this situation. They might be given feedback and instructions, coached and encouraged to rehearse more self-assertive behaviours. This kind of situation presented by Hersen *et al.* has come to be known in the literature as the 'unreasonable request'. It has been used extensively to assess general assertiveness, as a training exercise and also as an outcome measure in many studies (Hersen *et al.*, 1973; McFall and Marston, 1970). Many of the studies of assertion training have concentrated on what Wolpe (1969) called 'hostile assertive statements'. Wolpe, however, also drew attention to the need to help some patients make 'commendatory assertions', i.e. expressions of praise, approval, love and affection.

Much of the American research relevant to interpersonal skills training has focused on the refinement and evaluation of assertion training. Goldsmith and McFall (1975), on the basis of interviews with 74 psychiatric outpatients, identified seven situations that commonly gave rise to problems, and six aspects of interaction that were usually difficult for patients to handle. These are summarised in Table 2.1. Though they are drawn from a psychiatric outpatient population some of them may have a familiar ring to the reader as fairly common difficulties. Clearly, different groups of individuals undertaking particular social roles may also generate particular examples of difficulties of their own.

Table 2.1: Social Difficulty (Psychiatric Outpatients, USA)

Situations	Aspects of interaction
Dating	Initiating and terminating interactions
Making friends	Making personal disclosures
Having a job interview	Handling conversational silences
Relating to authority	Responding to rejection
Relating to service personnel	Being more self-assertive
Interacting with people perceived as more intelligent/ attractive	
Interacting with people whose appearance was different, e.g. race, physical handicap, etc.	

Source: After Goldsmith and McFall, 1975

These early developments in assertion training have made a number of important contributions to our understanding of some of the factors which need to be taken into account in looking at the development of interpersonal skills. Firstly, they have led to an awareness that there may often be an association between failures in self-assertion and the experience of psychological stress. Secondly, they draw attention to the need to consider positive assertiveness as important as negative assertion. A third contribution is the identification of a range of training components which can be used in putting together a training programme, e.g. modelling, rehearsal, etc. Fourthly, these developments draw attention to the need to identify particular situations or aspects of relationships that are a source of personal difficulty to the particular client group. These can then be made the focus of group training interventions.

Social Skills Training

In Britain the development of interpersonal skills training has been strongly influenced by the extensive research of social psychologists into the elements (verbal and non-verbal) of social performance. This research, together with the idea that the acquisition of socially skilled behaviour can be viewed as similar to the learning of any other skilled behaviour, has formed the basis of the approach advocated by Trower, Bryant and Argyle (1978). Psychologists who have concerned themselves with skilled human motor performance, have conceptualised it in terms of an integration of behaviours at a variety of different levels to produce smooth and co-ordinated responses to a changing situation. Training usually involves a preliminary analysis of the complex behaviour into the various levels of subskills of which it is constituted. Trainers proceed by devising ways of enabling trainees to practise the various subskills at each level before attempting to combine them into more complex sequences. According to Trower *et al.* this kind of analysis can be applied usefully to social behaviour. If we consider what is involved in refusing an unreasonable request from this point of view, we would tend to see it as a very complex piece of behaviour. This complex can be thought of as composed of a whole range of subskills. At the most basic level, components such as eye contact, facial expression, intonation, etc. can be identified. These basic elements, each of which might be performed in a way which is more or less effective, can be seen as being organised into more complex sequences such as 'listening' and 'speaking'. These sequences in turn can be regarded as being embedded in more complex patterns such as 'greeting people', 'apologising' or, as in our example, 'refusing an unreasonable request'. Viewing things in this way, a logical approach to interpersonal skills training is to carry out a careful practical pre-training assessment of the kinds of deficiencies that exist at different levels of skill. The trainee can then be taken through an individually designed programme which focuses on specific deficits. The programme should also help the trainee to integrate improved or newly developed subskills into a smooth performance.

Implications for Training Programmes

The SST approach is based on a 'curriculum model' and uses a much more detailed, step-by-step process of training than the American 'assertion training'. The approach used in assertion training has sometimes been called a 'situations approach', in that trainers using this approach tend to place an emphasis on role-played responses to real life situations from the outset. In a social skills 'curriculum approach', conversational role-plays may be set up for the specific purpose of improving a particular subskill. So posture or gesture may be worked on for a time before anything more complex is attempted. This approach makes intuitive sense when working with chronic psychiatric patients in whom even very basic social behaviour, such as eye contact, may be deficient. It might seem that this fine-grained approach is less appropriate when working with people who are generally more socially skilled, e.g. doctors or nurses. Even here however, in looking at particular areas of skill, such as 'interviewing patients', it may be useful to draw attention to the role of factors such as eye contact, posture etc. in establishing a good relationship. One thing which 'curriculum' and 'situations' approaches have in common is a similar selection of ingredients which go to make up the training programme.

Structure of Training Programmes

Underlying most social skills training programmes is an initial assessment phase, which might include amongst other things a simple role-play of a two or three person conversation. Once particular problems have been identified, they may be worked on systematically in a series of sessions. Each session might include any or all of the components shown in Table 2.2. Comparing these components with those used in assertion training it is clear that there is considerable overlap.

One other interesting conceptualisation which emerges from viewing socially skilled behaviour as similar to any other aspect of human skill, is the notion that skilled performance may break down at any one of its phases (see Figure 1.1). Thus, lack of goal clarity or inability to devise an appropriate strategy may lead to confusing or dissatisfying interactions; inadequate attention to external cues may lead to discord; and an inappropriate interpretative framework may dictate unfortunate social action. Assuming that relevant cues have been attended to and interpreted appropriately, a response must be planned. For many familiar day-to-day situations there are 'blueprints' for action and little specific thought may be necessary. If, however, someone is in the process of acquiring new skills, or the situation is a novel one, greater conscious

Table 2.2: Components of Social Skills Training Programmes

(1) *Dry Run* — this is usually a simple role play in which the trainee is asked to behave in his/her accustomed way. This is often videotaped.

(2) *Feedback and Instruction* — trainees are given some information about their performance, usually focusing on positive aspects and particular deficits. They may also be given explicit instructions about things they should try to do.

(3) *Modelling* — trainees can be provided with a modelled example of more appropriate behaviour. Writers on social skills have always stressed the importance of a fairly close matching between the model's level of skill and the trainee's current level so that too great a gap in performance is avoided.

(4) *Rehearsal and coaching* — the trainee is given an opportunity for further role-played practice. Sometimes the trainer actively coaches the trainee during this phase, giving instructions in mid-performance. A sophisticated version of this occurs, where the trainer observes the trainee's performance from behind a one-way screen or on closed circuit television and gives instructions via an earpiece worn by the trainee.

(5) *Reinforcing positive aspects of performance* — usually throughout sessions and at the end the trainer will reinforce positive aspects of performance with social approval.

(6) *Homework assignments* — trainees are often given exercises to carry out in real social settings between sessions. This is designed to facilitate transfer of skills and trainees are often required to keep a record of this practice and to report back at the next session.

effort may be required in planning the response.

Like any other skilled behaviour, as new behaviours become incorporated into the individual's repertoire they become gradually smoother and more automated and require less conscious attention and planning. This is a factor that needs to be taken into account in any skills training programme. There will often be a phase where trainees feel awkward, and that their behaviour is unnatural. It is obviously important for the trainer to provide good emotional support during this phase. In any activity, we often find that the response we make is not quite the response we intended. When this occurs, it is usually taken as a sign that more work is needed to establish better control over responses. It is at this stage that lack of skills often manifests itself in what is *said* and *done*. Many aspects of skill require good timing and this is also something that often needs to be worked on. Although all these issues are of acknowledged importance, sometimes too much emphasis has been given to 'executing responses' or social performance aspects, at the expense of cognitive aspects of social interaction.

Cognitive Aspects of Skilled Social Performance

An important consideration, though one that is sometimes not taken into account by social skills trainers, is that in order to behave in a skilled way it is necessary to have some degree of confidence in our ability to do so. Many authors have speculated about the complex relationship between cognitive self-appraisal and behaviour. Bandura (1977) has elaborated the concept of 'self-efficacy'. He argues that possessing a skill or competence does not necessarily lead to its use. Whether it is used or not depends to some extent on a cognitive factor, a belief in our capacity to perform effectively. This is what Bandura calls the person's sense of 'self-efficacy'. In many situations, people who possess skills also hold negative beliefs about their abilities which prevent them from using the skills they have. According to Bandura, individuals' sense of 'self-efficacy' will influence the extent to which they initiate behaviour. It will also influence their choice or avoidance of particular behavioural settings. Finally, it will influence their persistence. If we have a strong sense of 'self-efficacy' we are likely to try harder and for longer when we encounter difficulties. Within this formulation, people who appear to be deficient in social skills may not lack the appropriate responses, they may also hold the expectation that the response envisaged would be well received: what they may lack, however, is a sense of their own capacity to act in the desired way.

Bandura's model for promoting change, derived from these theoretical speculations, does not involve approaching the person's beliefs directly. Rather, he suggests an indirect approach via behaviour. Bandura argues that it is possible to give the individual experience of successful outcomes by prolonged exposure to graded modelling, using guided and reinforced imitation, in a situation where anxiety is kept within tolerable limits. If the learning situation is organised so that these outcomes can be experienced over an increasingly wider range of tasks, a sense of 'self-efficacy' is developed. 'Self-efficacy', according to Bandura, has the useful function of inoculating people against occasional setbacks.

This view appears to bear some resemblance to the 'inoculation' techniques advocated by Meichenbaum and Cameron (1973) and Seligman (1975), and also the notion of 'internal locus of control' put forward by Rotter (1966). It would appear that behaviour and cognitive self-appraisal are often locked together in a negative self-fulfilling prophecy. The trainer or therapist's role is to break into this self-fulfilling cycle. For some clients the appropriate approach may be a cognitive one, for others it may be behavioural or a combination of both. These considerations have led to an increasing interest in, and awareness of, the role of cognitive factors in social skills training. Heimberg and Becker (1981) draw attention to the importance of the kinds of things that people say to themselves (self-statements) when faced with difficult social interactions. Some statements seem to facilitate assertive responses and are referred to as positive. Others seem to inhibit self-assertion and are referred to as negative. For example, in response to an unreasonable request, the self-statement 'I have a right to refuse' tends to facilitate assertiveness. On the other hand a self-statement such as 'he/she will not like me if I refuse' will tend to undermine self-assertion. Schwartz and Gottman (1976) have developed an Assertion Self-Statement Test, and studies using this test have found differences in the distribution of positive and negative self-statements between assertive and non-assertive people. Assertive people tend to have predominantly positive self-statements, whereas non-assertive people reveal a mixture of positive and negative self-statements. It is as if non-assertive persons are experiencing an internal dialogue of conflict.

Ellis (1962) has discussed the role of irrational beliefs in maintaining dysfunctional behaviour patterns and has developed a method of therapy in which he systematically challenges these beliefs. Alden and Safran (1978) found that there was a correlation between holding irrational beliefs, such as 'I believe I should be competent at everything I attempt' and low levels of self-assertion. Both self esteem and internal locus of control were found by Spence and Spence (1980) and Kagan (1981) to be enhanced as a result of social skills training. In neither instance, though, could the changes be confidently attributed to the training itself, rather than to 'non-intended treatment effects'. Other studies have looked at the sorts of outcomes the person expects to result from more assertive or skilled performance. In a study by Fiedler and Beach (1978), subjects did not differ in their definition of particular outcomes as positive or negative, but did differ in their expectations that assertiveness would lead to positive rather than negative outcomes. Subjects who were more assertive expected assertiveness to produce positive outcomes and compliance negative ones. Subjects who were less assertive believed the reverse. Attempts have been made to develop an integrated behavioural and cognitive approach to training in which clients rehearse more effective behaviours but are also encouraged to examine and change their own internal thoughts and self-beliefs concerning interpersonal effectiveness. These issues are of relevance to nurses, if it is to be argued that lack of use of skill may not be due to lack of skill *per se* (see Chapter 3).

The Use of Videotape Recordings

Another feature of social skills training has been the extensive use which has been made of videotape recordings. Recordings have been used in four different ways.

Assessment. Role-played interactions are generally used, in which trainees are asked to behave as closely as possible to their normal pattern. These recordings can then be used as a basis for making an assessment of the areas of skill which need to be worked on. Clearly, role-playing in front of a camera can inject a degree of stress into a situation and also create a degree of artificiality which needs to be taken into account in any assessment. These tape recordings can be discussed with the trainee, and in this way allowances can be made for aspects of behaviour which result from role-playing in front of the camera. Assessment videotapes, made at intervals during training can provide useful benchmarks against which to assess change.

Models. It is useful to use videotaped role models to assist trainees. The literature has stressed how important it is that there should not be a big discrepancy between the role model and the trainee's own current level of skill. It is often therefore a good idea to use other trainees who are a little more advanced for modelling. The Communication in Patient Care material offers examples of good and bad models in different nursing settings (Hunt *et al.*, 1981).

Feedback. It is often very difficult to explain to someone the precise ways in which their behaviour in a situation is deficient. The use of videotaped feedback can facilitate the trainees' understanding of what may be going wrong and help them to make more appropriate responses to a situation. This can be done in a very supportive way by talking them through their behaviour. It is often useful to get them, themselves, to identify weaknesses in their handling of the situation, as they watch themselves on screen. Obviously someone whose skills are at a low level can easily be demoralised by seeing their poor performance on screen. This is therefore something that needs to be handled with tact and care by the trainer.

Self-training. Before undertaking skills training with any group, it is useful for any team or trainer(s) to go through a period of self-training, in which they can practise the various techniques outlined. This self-training not only allows the members of the team to gain confidence and skill in implementing the various procedures, but also gives them some insight into what it is like to be a trainee in this model. This is very important for the development of sensitivity in handling trainees' problems. Clearly, videotape can be a valuable part of this self-training exercise, providing useful feedback to trainers and also helping them to become less anxious and self-conscious about being on camera. If trainers are anxious about being filmed and having their behaviour monitored, they are quite likely to communicate this to their own trainees. When using videotape feedback, it is essential that some attention is paid to the possibility that participants may become very distressed (see Hung & Rosenthal (1978) for a review of the use of videotape recordings in psychotherapeutic settings, and Buss (1980) for a discussion of individual reactions to becoming objectively aware of 'self'). Careful monitoring and guidance by the trainer when viewing the tapes will usually overcome the anxieties, but it must be recognised that there is sometimes the need to dissipate anxiety that has been aroused.

Summary

To summarise briefly, social skills training has contributed to the development of interpersonal skills in a number of ways. Firstly, this work has drawn attention to the different levels of verbal and non-verbal skills and subskills involved in any complex social behaviour. From this point of view any training programme must identify deficiencies in skills and subskills, foster the development of these skills and create the conditions in which these subskills can become integrated into a smooth performance. Secondly, as with the work on assertion training, a series of training components has been identified which can be used in a skills programme. A third contribution, is the view that skills can break down at a number of stages and that it is important to establish at what point particular aspects of skill are breaking down, in order to make an appropriate intervention. A poor interviewer may be someone who does not have clear or appropriate goals, does not notice important cues from his/her client, misinterprets such cues, has difficulty in formulating appropriate responses, performs appropriate responses badly or is not receptive to feedback from the client. On the other hand, the person may be able to do all these things but in the real situation find him/

herself paralysed by worrying doubts about their own competence. Fourthly, this latter consideration has also led social skills trainers to an awareness of the importance of cognitive factors, although this is rarely incorporated, formally, into the training (Kagan, 1984). Finally, attention has been given to the many valuable ways in which closed circuit television and videotape recordings can contribute, in a carefully controlled and monitored way, to interpersonal skills training.

What are the Effective Components in Assertion and Social Skills Training Packages?

Many studies have been conducted in the psychiatric field in an attempt to identify the effective components of training packages. Different research designs have been used, the main distinction being between those which have used a group design with 'no training' or 'pseudo training' controls (e.g. McFall and Twentyman, 1973) and those which have used single case experimental designs (e.g. Hersen and Bellack, 1976b). The studies further subdivide into those which have investigated a full treatment programme, and 'analogue' studies which have used relatively short interventions with little or no follow up. Types of measures have included self-report, behavioural and psycho-physiological (especially in relation to anxiety); the behavioural measures have generally been based on role-plays and have included audio and videotaped assessments. Many of the early studies tried to assess short training programmes and rarely included follow-up studies; in addition the role-plays were often artificial, calling their validity into question. However, a number of conclusions about the effectiveness of different components of the training packages could be drawn. Generally, practice in the absence of instructions or coaching was relatively ineffective; coaching, rehearsal, feedback and, in some situations, modelling were all capable of producing strong treatment effects across a range of behavioural and self-report measures. Some combination of these elements, then, should provide the basis of any well constructed social skills package.

What Are the Best Ways to Measure the Progress and Outcome of Training Packages?

Attempts to assess the progress and outcome of social skills interventions seem to fall into three broad categories and it is worth examining these in some detail as they have implications for the monitoring and evaluation of any interpersonal skills training programme.

Standardised Inventories and Other Self-report Measures

A wide range of different inventories has been used in many studies. Some are specific to SST or assertion training, such as 'Assertiveness' scales (Gambrill and Richey, 1975; Rathus, 1973; Wolpe and Lazarus, 1966); and 'Interpersonal Situation' inventories (Goldsmith and McFall, 1975; Trower *et al.*, 1978). Others are of more general clinical application, and include the Taylor Manifest Anxiety Scale (see McFall and Marston, 1970), 'Social Anxiety and Distress', and 'Fear of Negative Evaluation' scales, developed by Watson and Friend (1969). Use of these scales has not been confined to clinical settings and they are currently being used in evaluations of training programmes for the Metropolitan Police Force and for bus drivers, amongst others!

To employ these types of scales as dependent measures has the advantage that in most instances they are of established reliability and validity in terms of their content. Unfortunately, a frequent outcome of their application to training programmes has been small non-significant changes or changes of a low order of significance. The difficulty in assessing the implications of these results for social skills training hinges on the fact that social skills training is directed towards producing a perceptible change in interaction behaviour, but even the best of these measures, designed with assertion or social skills in mind, provide only an indirect measure of actual interaction behaviour. Hersen and others have drawn attention to the cognitive lag which exists between behavioural change and subjective self-appraisal. Given the specific nature of much social skills behaviour, it has to be borne in mind that these general and self-report measures of performance and mood may fail to detect important behavioural changes.

Perhaps the most valuable kind of subjective measure is the one which seeks to establish whether the treatment package has altered the way in which individual clients conceptualise themselves. In this way one is at least able to evaluate the impact of the intervention on the client's self-conceptualisation irrespective of overt behavioural change. Repertory Grids (Fransella and Bannister, 1977; Kelly, 1955) provide one of the best tools in this direction. Appropriately designed grids can enable trainers and trainees to look at how the clients evaluate their own behaviour across a range of situations using their own constructs. Because the repertory grid technique was devised for measuring changes in individuals using their own constructs, it can provide a very sensitive measure of cognitive change in terms of variables that are subjectively relevant to the people themselves. A number of recent studies of the impact of professional training in the caring professions have used the repertory grid as a measure of subjective personal change (Heyman, Shaw and Harding, 1983; Liftshitz, 1974; Ryle and Breen, 1974).

Behavioural Tests

It follows from the arguments above that behavioural observations may provide better measures of the success or failure of a social skills intervention, and most research studies have included a measure of this type. McFall and Marston (1970) made use of a Behaviour Role-playing test. Sixteen stimulus situations requiring assertive responses were presented on audio tape. Responses to these were rated by independent raters for overall assertiveness. Later, Goldsmith and McFall (1975) developed the Interpersonal Behavior Role-playing Test, still designed to be presented on audio tape, but incorporating a wider range of situations. Eisler *et al.* (1975) developed the Behavioral Assertiveness Test along similar lines to McFall and Marston. The main difference was that clients had to interact with a confederate after each scene had been presented, and responses were videotaped. These tapes were rated on a number of non-verbal, negative-content and positive-content items, which had been found to differentiate between high and low assertive people using the Wolpe-Lazarus Assertiveness scale. Particularly significant variables were the length of speech, speech volume and number of speech disturbances. High assertive people requested more change in the behaviour of their role partners, complied less frequently, gave more praise and showed more positive spontaneous behaviours. Marzillier and Winter (1978) used the standard situation advocated by Trower *et al.* (1978) and rated subjects on specific individual behavioural targets, for example, amount of speech, hesitations, etc. They present no data on the reliability of their rating, but McFall and Eisler and Hersen all claim high reliability coefficients when using experienced raters.

The main defect of the McFall method seems to be the lack of a visual element in the assessment and the absence of a role partner. Eisler *et al.* (1975) remedied this defect in their study, but unfortunately the assessment scenes were, in most instances, the same scenes, in exactly the same format, as the ones used during the training phase. Although Hersen incorporated 'generalisation scenes' in some studies, these again were presented in precisely the same format and had very similar content to the rehearsal scenes. The identical nature both in form and content of training and assessment procedures in these studies seriously undermines the value to be placed on these assessments in terms of what they may tell us about behaviour outside the training situation.

Although the kinds of behavioural measures outlined above may appear to have high face validity, Cipani (1982) points out that empirical data concerning the validity of these measures, in terms of behaviour in naturally occurring situations, is sparse. It has been argued that the value of role-played behavioural tests can be increased by attention to a number of factors. Eisler (1976) emphasised the need to make role-playing scenes as vivid as possible, to use a variety of scenes in order to obtain a broad sample of the clients' social skills and to arrange for observers to be as unobtrusive as possible.

In Vivo *Assessment*

Since one of the main aims of social skills training is to produce lasting changes in everyday behaviour, there has been considerable interest in developing *in vivo* measures of social skills. Hersen, Eisler and Miller (1974) promised participants in their study a financial reward of $3 for completing the course. At the end of the programme participants were short-changed, being given only $1. Their reactions to this were videotaped and analysed for latency of response and overall assertiveness. Kazdin (1974) made use of a 'telephone follow-up', a device which had been used by McFall. Typically clients are telephoned after completion of the study by a confederate acting the role of, for example, a salesman who puts pressure on the client to purchase materials. Clients are rated in terms of their ability to resist these demands. In the McFall study, not all the participants were taken in by the phoney salesman, and others thought the demands being made were reasonable. Gutride, Goldstein and Hunter (1973), who were researching on a psychiatric inpatient population, had raters observe the behaviour of clients during mealtimes as part of their post-training procedures. Self-report measures of *in vivo* behaviour have been used by Marzillier and others. Clients have been asked to keep social diaries. Trower *et al.* (1978) present an interview schedule in which a range of social activities, social contacts and frequency of social behaviour is explored.

On the whole, attempts at assessment *in vivo*, whilst a necessary part of evaluating a training programme, are fraught with problems. *In vivo* behavioural assessments present difficulties in unobtrusive recording and standardisation. Given these difficulties, many studies have preferred to use the simpler and less expensive expedient of self-reporting, preferring to gamble on the honesty of subjects rather than indulge in the elaborate subterfuge of some of the American studies, and thus they avoid the ethical problems of deception. Professional training situations, however, possibly offer different opportunities for *in vivo* measurement. The keeping of detailed diaries of interactions and their outcome is clearly a useful feature of any training programme at whatever level.

Does Training Have Long Term Effects and Generalise to Other Situations?

The original analogue studies of skill training were of short term duration and were therefore unable to assess long-term effects. They also did not include specific tests to determine whether skills generalised to situations other than those used in training. Both of these issues have been recognised as crucial in establishing the efficacy of social skills training. Hersen and Bellack (1976a) have also argued that it is important not to confuse the two.

Bellack *et al.* (1976) tried to incorporate both features in an experiment with three chronic psychiatric patients in which they made use of three sets of eight scenes. One set was used for training, one set as probes for generalisation, administered at intervals during the course of training, and the third set used at intervals during an eight-week follow-up. The results from this study showed good generalisation and follow-up effects. It has been pointed out, however, that there are two ways of approaching the problems of generalisation. One is to use probe scenes similar in content and format to the original training scenes. This has been done extensively by Hersen, Eisler and Miller (1974). On the whole, these studies tend to show good generalisation effects. Studies which have attempted to demonstrate generalisation or transfer from structured training items to related but different situations in real life have been less successful. The studies quoted in the previous section, which have incorporated various *in vivo* measurement procedures have generally produced disappointing results. In discussing this, Eisler, Hersen, Miller and Blanchard (1975) and Goldsmith and McFall (1975) refer to Mischel's views on the context-specific nature of human behaviour:

> Response patterns even in highly similar situations often fail to be
> strongly related. Individuals show far less cross-situational consis-
> tency in their behaviour than has been assumed by trait-state
> theories. (Mischel, 1968, p.177)

Heimberg and Becker (1981) point out that this idea that behaviour
is highly specific to particular situations has been a strong theme in
interpersonal skills research. It has tended to replace earlier ideas that
characteristics such as assertiveness are generalised traits. Eisler *et al.*
(1975) were able to demonstrate this in one study. They showed that
variations in the sex or familiarity of the role partner, and in the nature
of the response required (positive or negative assertion), had implications for a diverse range of response variables including length of
speech, amount of smiling, amount of eye contact, etc. They were also
able to demonstrate complex interaction effects between the three variables. Heimberg and Becker (1981) claim that their data indicate that
this specific influence of situational variables becomes stronger as the
complexity of the task increases. Attribution theorists have argued that
in developing explanations of other people's behaviour most of us
exhibit what they call the 'fundamental attribution error' (Ross, 1977).
That is to say, we tend to favour 'trait' explanations when, often, a
situational explanation would be more appropriate. The research into
social skills seems to confirm this tendency to de-emphasise the power
of situations as determinants of behaviour. It suggests that in any interventions designed to produce more than specific responses to particular
situations, attention needs to be paid to the many ways in which situations vary, e.g. sex of the person we are interacting with, setting, etc.
These important variations need to be integrated into the training programme. That is, skill does not reside in the person, but is partly determined by other people and the environment.

Another general theoretical issue which has a bearing on generalisation is 'response class independence'. It has been pointed out that there
is considerable evidence that the various response classes which make
up assertive behaviour are relatively independent of each other (Heimberg and Becker, 1981), thus classes of behaviour only show improvement when specifically targeted in the training programme. So, for
example, working on a component like eye contact does not tend to produce improvements in other components such as posture. Similarly, at
a more molar level, work on negative assertion for example, does not
necessarily produce improvements in positive assertiveness. Lawrence
(1970) found that training subjects to disagree with others' opinions did

not improve their ability to agree with opinions they found compatible. These findings indicate that in order to establish generalisation, it is important not only to pay attention to situational variations but also to the different classes of behaviour which are required. Training for generalisation, then, requires careful attention to situational variables and response variables, and an effort to include an appropriate range of these into training programmes.

One component of social skills training which may well facilitate generalisation is the formulation of specific homework goals that draw attention to situation variables and specific practice points. Shepherd (1978) reports some success with these techniques. He emphasises the need for detailed goal setting, and Hersen and Bellack (1976a) discuss the value of cognitive self-regulation in facilitating generalisation and advocate self-monitoring, self-evaluation and self-reinforcement techniques. Meichenbaum (1977) has also discussed the value of these kinds of self-regulatory behaviours in improving existing behavioural treatments.

The research on psychiatric populations suggests that generalisation of the effects of training across situations and behaviours and long-term effects cannot be assumed, and there is no reason to suppose that nursing settings are different. Thought needs to be given, in the design of programmes, to how generalisation is to be achieved. Simply instructing trainees to do this appears not to work, although following the trainees through into the practical situation and providing suitable prompts seems to help. This has implications for nurse tutor/clinical nursing relationships (see Bill Reynolds, Chapter 14). Due regard needs to be paid to the many ways in which situations vary and the many specific behaviours that comprise a skilled performance in those different situations. As wide a range of these factors as possible needs to be built into the training programe. As far as long-term effects are concerned, it is probably safest to regard all changes in behaviour as likely to be short term, unless followed up in some way. Perhaps we should regard professional training in interpersonal skills as continuous rather than something which happens at a particular point in time.

Postscript

So far, a model of interpersonal skills is emerging which sees skilled behaviour as a result of a complex interaction between *emotional* factors, such as level of anxiety, *skill* factors, such as possessing appropriate behaviours or accurately perceiving cues, and *cognitive* factors, such as beliefs about oneself and one's competence. These variables are seen to be brought into play in particular situations which make their own particular demands on the participants' repertoires of available responses. One assumption that has been built into this model (Heimberg and Becker, 1981) is that if more assertive or skilled responses occur, other participants in the situation will respond favourably, thus reinforcing more assertive and skilled behaviour. Research studies reviewed by Heimberg, however, suggest that this may not necessarily be the case. Hollandsworth and Cooley (1978) and Mullinix and Galassi (1981) found that while assertion was preferred to aggression, it did not emerge as necessarily preferred to non-assertive behaviour. Woolfolk and Dever (1979) found that assertive behaviour was rated as less polite, more hostile and less satisfying to the recipient than non-assertive behaviour. Kelly, Kern, Kirkley, Patterson and Keane (1980) found that actors performing more assertively were perceived as more skilled and able, but less likeable, than actors performing passively. Kelly *et al.* (1980) also found that assertive behaviour was evaluated more negatively in females than in males behaving in the same way. While it is appropriate to be concerned with improving the interpersonal skills and assertiveness of individuals, we must not ignore the influence of other people present, and of the powerful situational variables demanding specific behaviour that may be judged to be unskilled. Thus it may be made difficult for patients to be appropriately assertive and express their own views about how much or how little information and help they would like. Similarly, strong nursing and medical hierarchies may dictate the amount of information a nurse at a specific level may reveal or the extent to which she/he may (acceptably) be assertive. If particular individuals or groups operating in such a hierarchy develop their skills, they may find that they are transgressing a situational norm (see Chapters 3, 4 and 5 for further discussion of these themes). Any attempt to improve the social skills of particular individuals must also be accompanied by efforts to improve social environments, so that more skilled and assertive behaviours are widely valued by all the participants.

References

Alden, L. and Safran, J.D. (1978) 'Irrational Beliefs and Non-assertive Behavior', *Cognitive Therapy and Research*, 2, 357-64

Argyle, M. (ed.) (1981a) *Social Skills and Work*, Methuen: London

Argyle, M. (ed.) (1981b) *Social Skills and Health*, Methuen: London

Bandura, A. (1977) 'Self-Efficacy: Towards a unifying theory of behavioral change', *Psychological Review*, 84, 191-215

Bellack, A.S., Hersen, M. and Turner, S.M. (1976) 'Generalisation Effects of Social Skills Training in Chronic Schizophrenics: An experimental analysis', *Behaviour Research and Therapy*, 14, 391-7

Buss, A.H. (1980) *Self Consciousness and Social Anxiety*, Freeman: San Francisco

Cipani, E. (1982) 'Social Skills Training with Institutionalised Clients: A critical review', *Corrective and Social Psychiatry and Journal of Behavior Technology*, 28, 31-40

Davidson, C. (1980) 'The Introduction and Evaluation of a Social Skills Training Programme on a Psychiatric In-patient Unit', unpublished MSc thesis: Leeds University

Eisler, R.M. (1976) 'Behavioral Assessment of Social Skills' in M. Hersen and A.S. Bellack (eds), *Behavioral Assessment: A practical handbook*, Pergamon Press: New York

Eisler, R.M., Hersen, M., Miller, P.M. and Blanchard, E.B. (1975) 'Situational Determinants of Assertive Behaviors', *Journal of Consulting and Clinical Psychology*, 43, 330-40

Ellis, A. (1962) *Reason and Emotion in Psycho-therapy*, Stuart: New York

Ellis, R.A.F. and Whittington, D. (1981) *A Guide to Social Skill Training*, Croom Helm: London

Fiedler D. and Beach, L.R. (1978) 'On the Decision to be Assertive', *Journal of Consulting and Clinical Psychology*, 46, 537-46

Fransella, F. and Bannister, D. (1977) *A Manual for Repertory Grid Technique*, Academic Press: London

Friedman, P.M. (1971) 'The Effects of Modelling and Role Playing on Assertive Behavior' in R.B. Rubin, H. Fernsterheim and A. Lazarus (eds) *Advances in Behavior Therapy*, Academic Press: New York

Gambrill, E.D. and Richey, C.A. (1975) 'An Assertion Inventory for Use in Assessment and Research', *Behavior Therapy*, 6, 550-61

Goldsmith, J.B. and McFall, R.M. (1975) 'Development and Evaluation of an Interpersonal Skill Training Programme for Psychiatric In-patients', *Journal of Abnormal Psychology*, 54, 51-8

Gutride, M.E., Goldstein, A.P. and Hunter, G.R. (1973) 'The Use of Modelling and Role Playing to Increase Social Interaction among Asocial Psychiatric Patients', *Journal of Consulting and Clinical Psychology*, 40, 408-15

Heimberg, R.G. and Becker, R.E. (1981) 'Cognitive and Behavioral Models of Assertive Behavior: Review, analysis and integration', *Clinical Psychology Review*, 1, 353-73

Hersen, M. and Bellack, A.S. (1976a) 'Social Skills Training for Chronic Psychiatric Patients: Rationale, research findings and future directions', *Comprehensive Psychiatry*, 17, 559-80

Hersen, M. and Bellack, A.S. (1976b) 'A Multiple-Baseline Analysis of Social Skills Training in Chronic Schizophrenics', *Journal of Applied Behavior Analysis*, 9, 239-45

Hersen, M., Eisler, R.M. and Miller, P.M. (1973) 'Effects of Practice, Instructions and Modelling on Components of Assertive Behaviour', *Behaviour Research and Therapy*, 11, 443-51

Hersen, M., Eisler, R.M. and Miller, P.M. (1974) 'An Experimental Analysis of Generalisation in Assertive Training', *Behaviour Research and Therapy*, *12*, 295-310

Heyman, R., Shaw, M.P. and Harding, J. (1983) 'A Personal Construct Theory Approach to the Socialisation of Nursing Trainees in Two British General Hospitals', *Journal of Advanced Nursing*, *8*, 59-67

Hollandsworth, J.G. and Cooley, M.L. (1978) 'Provoking Anger and Gaining Compliance with Assertive Versus Aggressive Responses', *Behavior Therapy*, *9*, 640-6

Hung, J.H.F. and Rosenthal, T.L. (1978) 'Therapeutic Videotaped Playback: A critical review', *Advances in Behaviour Research and Therapy*, *1*, 103-35

Hunt, J., Macleod Clark, J., Redfern, S. and Tippett, J. (eds) (1981) *Communication in Patient Care*, Project in Collaboration with The Kings Fund: Abbot Laboratories

Kagan, C. (1981) 'Cognitive Aspects of Social Skills Training', unpublished DPhil. thesis: University of Oxford

Kagan, C. (1984) 'Social Problem Solving and Social Skills Training', *British Journal of Clinical Psychology*, *23*, 161-73

Kazdin, A.E. (1974) 'Effects of Covert Modelling and Model Reinforcement on Assertive Behavior', *Journal Abnormal Psychology*, *83*, 240-52

Kelly, G.A. (1955) *The Psychology of Personal Constructs*, Vols. 1 & 2, Merton: New York

Kelly, J.A., Kern, J.M., Kirkley, B.G., Patterson, J.N. and Keane, T.M. (1980) 'Reactions to Assertive *v.* Unassertive Behavior. Differential Effects for Males and Females and Implications for Assertiveness Training', *Behavior Therapy*, *11*, 670-82

Lawrence, P.S. (1970) 'The Assessment and Modification of Assertive Behavior', Unpublished PhD Thesis: Arizona State University *Dissertation Abstracts International*, *31*, 396B

Liftshitz, M. (1974) 'Quality Professionals: Does training make a difference? A Personal Construct Theory Study of the Issue', *British Journal of Social and Clinical Psychology*, *13*, 183-9

Marzillier, J.S., Lambert, C. and Kellett, J. (1976) 'A Controlled Evaluation of Systematic Desensitisation and Social Skills Training for Socially Inadequate Psychiatric Patients', *Behaviour Research and Therapy*, *14*, 225-38

Marzillier, J.S. and Winter, K. (1978) 'Success and Failure in Social Skills Training: Individual differences', *Behaviour Research and Therapy*, *16*, 67-84

Meichenbaum, D. (1977) *Cognitive Behavior Modification: An Integrative Approach*, Plenum: New York

Meichenbaum, D. and Cameron, R. (1973) 'Stress Inoculation: A skills training approach to anxiety management', unpublished manuscript: University of Waterloo

McFall, R.M. and Lillesand, D.B. (1971) 'Behavior Rehearsal with Modelling and Coaching in Assertion Training', *Journal of Abnormal Psychology*, *77*, 313-23

McFall, R.M. and Marston, A.R. (1970) 'An Experimental Investigation of Behavior Rehearsal in Assertive Training', *Journal of Abnormal Psychology*, *76*, 295-303

McFall, R.M. and Twentyman, C.T. (1973) 'Four Experiments on the Relative Contribution of Rehearsal, Modelling and Coaching to Assertion Training', *Journal of Abnormal Psychology*, *81*, 199-218

Mischel, W. (1968) *Personality Assessment*, Wiley: New York

Mullinix, S.D. and Galassi, J.P. (1981) 'The Role of Social Perception in Social Skill', *Behavior Therapy*, *12*, 69-79

Rahe, R.H., Floistad, I., Bergan, T., Ringdal, R., Gerhardt, R., Gunderson, E.K.E. and Arthur, R.J. (1974) 'A Model for Life Changes and Illness Research', *Archives of General Psychiatry*, *31*, 172-7

Rathus, S.A. (1973) 'A 30-item Schedule for Assessing Assertive Behavior', *Behavior Therapy*, *4*, 398-406

Ross, L. (1977) 'The Intuitive Psychologist and his Shortcomings: Distortions in the Attribution Process', in L. Berkowitz (ed.), *Advances in Experimental Social Psychology*, *10*, Academic Press: New York

Rotter, J.B. (1966) 'Generalised Expectancies for Internal versus External Control of Reinforcement', *Psychological Monographs: General and Applied*, *80*, 1-27

Ryle, A. and Breen, D. (1974) 'Changes in the Course of Social Work Training: A repertory grid study', *British Journal of Medical Psychology*, *47*, 139

Schwartz, R.M. and Gottman, J.M. (1976) 'Toward a Task Analysis of Assertive Behavior', *Journal of Consulting and Clinical Psychology*, *44*, 910-20

Seligman, M.E.P. (1975) *Helplessness,* Freeman: San Francisco

Shepherd, G. (1978) 'Social Skills Training: The generalisation problem — some further data', *Behaviour Research and Therapy*, *16*, 287-8

Spence, A.J. and Spence, S.H. (1980) 'Cognitive Changes Associated with Social Skills Training', *Behaviour Research and Therapy*, *18*, 265-72

Trower, P.E., Bryant B. and Argyle, M. (1978) *Social Skills and Mental Health*, Methuen: London

Watson, D. and Friend, R. (1969) 'Measurement of Social-Evaluative Anxiety', *Journal of Consulting and Clinical Psychology*, *33*, 448-57

Wilkinson, J. and Canter, S. (1982) *Social Skills Training Manual*, Wiley: London

Wolpe, J. (1969) *The Practice of Behavior Therapy*, Pergamon: New York

Wolpe, J. and Lazarus, A.A. (1966) *Behavior Therapy Techniques*, Pergamon: New York

Woolfolk, R.L. and Dever, S. (1979) 'Perceptions of Assertion: An empirical analysis', *Behavior Therapy*, *10*, 404-11

3 THE NEED FOR RESEARCH INTO INTERPERSONAL SKILLS IN NURSING

Peter Banister and Carolyn Kagan

Introduction

It is not unusual for people working both in and out of the health field to consider that interpersonal skills (IPS) are a matter of common sense and occur naturally. Friedman and DiMatteo (1982, p.6) point out that many health care professionals (including nurses) feel that the

> . . . interpersonal issues involved in practitioner-patient interactions are naturally and automatically understood and acted upon. Many practitioners believe that interpersonal issues do not require active concern and scientific study.

These views are echoed by French (1983, p.9), who notes that

> . . . there is still a common belief that socially skilled action and methods of interpersonal relating are not amenable to training or education. It is still common to hear nurses at all levels say that social skills just come naturally.

In order to make a case for the need to do research into IPS in nursing, and bring it out of the 'common sense' and into the 'scientific' domain, it is necessary to address several issues: (1) the identification of IPS: what *are* they? What is *interpersonal* about them? and what does it mean to refer to them as *skills*? (2) the identification of IPS in *nursing*: do they differ from IPS in any other context(s)? Who decides what the skills should be? And how are these decisions implemented in the context of contemporary policy? (3) the thorny question of why do research into practical nursing anyway? What kind of research is most appropriate to nurses? And what does and should happen to the research findings?

Discussion of most of these issues will take place in subsequent chapters, but this chapter will attempt an overview, and highlight what may be seen to be some of the most relevant themes.

The Nature of Interpersonal Skills

It could be argued that almost everything nurses do is interpersonal, in that it is in conjunction with at least one other person. However, nursing has traditionally been seen to be ' . . . almost exclusively care-oriented following the medical model of disease, with an emphasis on institutional care concerned with acute episodes of illness' (Crow, 1982, p.37). This has meant that the social aspects of nursing have been subjugated to the task aspects. IPS refer to the social and affective (or emotional) features of nursing care, rather than to the manual, technical features. To refer to these activities as skills, however, is to use a metaphor from the technical field, a metaphor that has been used in this country for several years in the context of general social interaction skills (Argyle, 1969, 1982; Argyle and Kendon, 1967).

There are several features of skills that are worth mentioning for the implications they have for IPS in nursing. The first, and perhaps the most important for dispelling the belief about the 'common sense' basis, is that they are *learnt*. Furthermore, they can nearly always be improved upon, or developed. Just as they can be learnt well, so they can be learnt poorly: good IPS are due to successful learning (and can, potentially, be modified to become less good), and poor IPS are due to unsuccessful learning (and can, potentially, be modified to become better). Thus the second feature is that, in order to maintain a high level of skill, it is necessary to *practise*. Skills are usually complex, and the third feature of a skill is that it can be broken down into identifiable *components or stages* that, combined, produce the overall skill. The fourth feature is that if skills are learnt, they *can also be taught*, preferably through demonstration, guidance (practice) and feedback.

One consequence of adopting a skills approach to IPS in nursing has been writers claiming that IPS in nursing care are, indeed, learnt (Macleod Clark, 1981a), must be practised (Davis, 1981a) and can be taught (Davis 1982; Faulkner and Maguire, 1984). Furthermore, some of the components of effective skills for nurses have been identified (see for example the various chapters in Bridge and Macleod Clark (1981) which emphasise the different skills required in specific nursing contexts).

Identification of Interpersonal Skills in Nursing

Nursing differs substantially from other interaction contexts, owing to the particular characteristics of patients, nurses and the nursing context. Patients may behave in unpredictable ways that bear little resemblance to their usual social behaviour outside the patient role. Most basically, patients are ill. Their illness may be distressing, painful, distorting of senses such as sight, hearing, touch and even consciousness. These factors may all result in increased emotionality and perceived (di)stress. Parsons (1951) drew attention to the 'sick role' adopted by, or imposed upon, patients. Medical and nursing personnel help construct the role which allows patients to abdicate their normal social responsibilities, and exempts them from responsibility for their condition, whilst at the same time obliging them to cooperate in order to get well. Thus the 'good' patients are the conforming ones who do exactly what is expected of them, even before coming to hospital (Roberts, 1984), and by so doing legitimate the nursing role (Kelly and May, 1982). Whether or not the model of the 'sick role' is adopted, a major illness or operation must be seen to constitute a 'life event', which will itself contribute to feelings of stress, and may even exacerbate the illness (Rabkin and Struening, 1976).

There are other dimensions to the experience of life as a patient that may contribute to perceived stress. Lack of control over physical resources, such as temperature, furniture, personal possessions, even food (Kagan and Burton, 1982), and associated with this, lack of decision-making opportunities (Orford, 1981), may all lead to feelings of frustration and distress. As patients experience lack of success in gaining control over these resources or decisions, due largely to institutional rules or regulations or practices, they may well succumb to a state of apathy and not even bother to try any longer: in some cases, this apathy may lead to depression. All these reactions characterise what Barton (1976) terms 'institutional neurosis', and are particularly prevalent in 'total institutions' (Goffman, 1961), wherein all the activities of daily living are carried out in the same place — the ward for instance. (For a critical discussion of these notions see Orford, 1981.)

Not all patients will respond in the same way to their role, and there are vast individual differences in response to stress (Clarke, 1984). As noted above, apathy and depression are rife, but so is a more aggressive demandingness. The different responses from patients precipitate different attitudes from nurses (and possibly behaviour, though this has not been demonstrated) (Kelly and May, 1982). Stockwell (1972) was the first to note that patients who ask a lot of questions become unpopular. It is not surprising that they persist in their questioning when, as Rosenhan (1973) showed, only 6 per cent of questions asked by patients of (admittedly) psychiatrists elicited any verbal response whatsoever.

Nurses, too, in their role, may behave differently from in other spheres of their lives. The context in which they work (including tasks, rules and regulations, the physical environment, as well as the wider social/political context and the other people involved) defines, to a large extent, the behaviours expected of them. Murray (1983) suggests that one reason nurses decide to leave the profession is because of the conflict they experience between their self-image and what they perceive to be the public's expectations of them. The public includes patients. First year student nurses do not experience this conflict as, he suggests, they have not yet become fully aware of the public's demands. As they do become aware of these demands, student nurses begin to experience the conflict. This study, whilst raising an interesting issue, begs the question of whether the public *does* have — and express — unrealistic expectations of nurses, or whether nurses simply *perceive* it to be so. Either way, the consequence is perceived role conflict and dissatisfaction with nursing. Other distinctive features of the nurses' role are those that relate to the ethical and moral issues they are often forced to confront. For nurses to work with patients who have attempted suicide, had abortions, are undergoing electro-convulsive shock treatment and so on, when they, themselves hold strong moral and ethical (and sometimes religious) views, may contribute to considerable role strain. Not all such dilemmas are in the nurses' power to reconcile. Take, for example, the question of whether or not patients (should) have the right to know fully about their own medical condition, an especially contentious issue if that condition is terminal (Hitch and Murgatroyd, 1983). Kelly and May (1982) point out that in such cases it is generally the medical profession that *defines* the nature of the nurse-patient relationship. Glaser and Strauss (1965) have suggested that the least stressful way of relating to terminally ill people is to do so in what they refer to as an 'open awareness' context. This is one where patient (or relative) and carer are both free and able to openly express and receive each other's fears and worries about the sick person's condition. Field (1984) reports nurses' accounts of nursing dying patients in an 'open disclosure' context, fully supported by senior medical and nursing staff on the ward. Most nurses preferred the open awareness context, but emphasised the importance of openness and flexibility in the ward routine, and such a supportave situation. Knight and Field (1981) argue that in a formal and hierarchical ward, open awareness would be difficult to achieve, and attempts to do so in the absence of personal support would be particularly stressful. Field's (1984) study is interesting in several ways. Firstly he notes that his findings are inconsistent with those of McIntosh (1977), just seven years earlier. McIntosh found that medical and nursing staff preferred a situation wherein the patients did not know of their condition, but the relatives did. The significance of this is that interpersonal issues in health care are not static, and that they change with shifts in policy, social attitudes and even as we shall see later, possibly as a direct result of the dissemination of earlier research findings. Secondly, Field suggests that the quality of communication between doctors and nurses is of critical importance. This view is upheld by Forgan-Morle's (1984) finding that elderly men and women made a point of stressing their dislike of the lack of communication between doctors and nurses. Finally, Field points to the importance of supportive networks in areas of nursing that are emotionally charged, and where nurses are encouraged to take responsibility for their relationships with patients. Clearly, if staff morale is low, effective communication will be distorted (Revans, 1964), or barriers will be erected in order to reduce the possibility of stress (e.g. Faulkner, 1981).

Several other writers have pointed to the essential role that personal support for nurses plays (Macleod Clark, 1981b). McIntee and Firth (1984), in discussing the problem of 'burnout' for nurses, suggest that supportive communication with colleagues is vital in enabling staff to provide a good quality service. Altschul (1983), too, asserts that support systems will be essential if the profession is seriously interested in encouraging and facilitating more meaningful and therapeutic forms of communication between nurses and patients. Nurses will not be able to determine what the patients may reveal, and this could well turn out to be more distressing than anticipated. Indeed, the Royal College of Nursing (1978, p.16) acknowledges that ' . . . nursing has long been recognised as a profession in which personal and institutional stresses are inherent'.

In summary, it is stressful to be either patient or nurse, but for rather different reasons. This means that patient and nurse may well be communicating with each other in ways that are not typical of their usual ways of relating. This does not necessarily mean that they do not *possess the skills* of interaction, but rather that they may not be *using them* in the nursing context. This is a crucial issue for research into IPS in nursing, and one must take cognisance of this possibility when considering what questions to ask, and how to research them. We shall argue later that to look at nurses' behaviour in isolation from the physical, organisational and social context, may give a misleading picture of the complexity, and indeed the levels of 'skill' involved in the employment of IPS by nurses.

Definition of Appropriate Interpersonal Skills

Research into IPS in nursing cannot proceed without some recognition of what skills are necessary and desirable. Several official publications have outlined, in terms broad enough to be meaningless, the basic requirements for effective interpersonal skills.

The Briggs Report (1972, p.44) emphasised that the objectives of nursing included ' ... continuity and coordination of care in the interests of the comfort, recovery and integrity of the person being cared for'. It went on to stress that a major nursing skill is the prescription of an *appropriate social context* for treatment. Who decides what such an appropriate social context is? In a similar vein, the Royal College of Nursing (1978) announced that increased emphasis should be given to the development of *elementary communication and human relationship skills* in all types of nurse training. Is there something universal about elementary communication and human relationship skills? If not, who decides what they are? The GNC syllabus now recognises that the relationship between the nurse, patients and relatives; the place of the nurse in the hospital team; and relationships with other staff, should all be included in basic nurse training curricula. But *what* is it about these relationships that should be included, and who decides?

The answers to these questions might help in assessing the adequacy and value of existing research, in identifying research questions and in determining the most useful type of research to be conducted, in order to effect neccessary change.

The Nature of Research in Interpersonal Skills in Nursing

There is no doubt that the work on IPS in nursing has derived its impetus from well established research traditions in other fields. Academic social psychology, clinical and counselling psychology, sociology and, to a lesser extent, management psychology, have all contributed paradigms for conducting research and have helped to identify some 'desirable skills' that should, perhaps be aspired to. Working models for research (and training) have been based in the UK on, for example, the Social Skills model (after Argyle, 1969; Ellis and Whittington, 1981), and empathy training (after Carkhuff, 1969). In the USA, approaches have included those based on assertion training (after Wolpe, 1969), interpersonal process recall (IPR) (Kagan, 1975) and, again, empathy training. As so many different models are used, conceptual confusion is rife, and this increases the likelihood that ill-defined research questions will be asked, based on shaky rationale.

Macleod Clark (1983) notes with some surprise that despite all the dissemination of research findings demonstrating the importance of nurse-patient communication, nurses on surgical wards spent little time talking to patients. So it seems that clinical nurses are not using the research findings. Hunt (1984) suggests five reasons why this may be: they may not understand the findings; they may disbelieve the findings if they contradict their own assumptions; they may lack permission to put the findings into practice if this would mean changing established practices; or they may lack incentive, in so far as anything new is hard work! A further possibility is suggested by Greenwood (1984) who contends that clinical nurses do not perceive research findings as relevant to their clinical practice. This view is reiterated by Rank, Rostron and Stenhouse (1984), who suggest that a great deal of nursing research is descriptive and therefore impossible to implement — a comment that is particularly pertinent to research into IPS in nursing.

On the whole, the research is done 'on' nurses, rather than 'with' nurses, thereby treating the nurses as 'objects' to be studied. This approach has several consequences for the acceptance and utility of the findings. Firstly, the nurses may not feel involved at all, and may, therefore discount the findings as being of interest only to the researcher. Secondly, the nurses might not feel that the questions that were asked were the most important or relevant. Why not, then, *ask practising nurses what their problems with communication are*? Will this really detract from the objectivity that is so highly valued in the scientific field (Clark and Hockey, 1979)? Bond and Bond (1982) did ask clinical nurses what their research priorities were, and suggested a repeated survey technique, known as the Delphi technique, as a manageable way of doing this. Hitch and Murgatroyd (1983) criticise much of the work on communication in nursing for its emphasis on verbal communication: as a result of this, they claim

> . . . it is not possible to say whether nurses recognise that they have communication problems. There appears to be scant research directed at nurses' attitudes towards communication and its difficulties, nor more importantly, their views of what could be done to solve these problems. (Hitch and Murgatroyd, 1983, pp. 413-4)

This is an important point if it is the case, as we have suggested above, that nurses have interpersonal skills, but for various reasons do not use them. In their study, Hitch and Murgatroyd found that nurses were indeed able to identify some problems, and some administrative and educational solutions to these problems. There may be no need therefore to do the 'objective', fact-finding research 'on' the nurses — they could just be asked.

We have just suggested that one reason research findings in the field of IPS in nursing have not been adopted is due to the lack of involvement by clinical nurses in formulating the research questions. Clark and Hockey (1979, p.4) summarise the predominant view of research in nursing as follows: ' . . . research findings provide us with objectively determined factual knowledge, whereas previous experience provides us with subjective accumulation of intuitive knowledge.' This approach is essentially an empiricist one, and as such is subject to several shortcomings. We will argue that to adopt such a stance with regard to IPS is to (1) misunderstand the nature of social 'facts' (in relation, here, to interpersonal behaviour); (2) adopt a mechanistic and reductionist view of people, whereby any part of them can be legitimately studied in isolation from the whole person; and (3) suggest that people can be studied as 'objects' in the social world, rather than as 'subjects' that form, and are changed by, the social world.

Furthermore, such an approach leads to particular forms of research activity that have many methodological pitfalls, and these considerably reduce the practical utility of the findings.

The prevailing research paradigm in IPS in nursing can be challenged, therefore, with respect to the nature of individuals and social facts, and the validity of the research findings. We shall discuss these two themes, drawing considerably on theoretical and methodological critiques that have been developed in 'academic' social psychology.

The Nature of Individuals and Social Facts

During the 1970s, a theoretical debate raged concerning the relevance of social psychological investigations. Harré and Secord (1972), Israel and Tajfel (1972) and Armistead (1974) criticised research practices that dictated the control and isolation of variables about people or social behaviour. In other words, they criticised empiricist approaches to social behaviour. People were not, they asserted, passive objects to be studied like any other inert object: rather, they were active agents who changed and influenced their social environment and were, in turn, influenced by the very social environment they had created. Instead, these writers championed more humanistic approaches to people that would encourage the ' . . . reports of feelings, plans, intentions, beliefs, reasons and so on, (whereby) the meanings of social behaviour, and the rules underlying social acts can be discovered' (Harré and Secord, 1972, p.7). To adopt this view, would mean that researchers would have to involve their subjects fully in the research process, and continually 'check out' their own interpretation of their findings with their subjects.

Take, for example, the case of a researcher finding that nursing staff on the afternoon shift on an orthopaedic ward spent very little time talking to patients. What does this mean if:

(1) researcher asks nurses why they did not talk to the patients, and is told 'we're preoccupied with the recent (sudden) transfer of the Sister we really got on with: we're sure the Consultant has complained about her'; or

(2) researcher asks nurses why they did not talk to the patients and is told 'we couldn't be bothered'; or

(3) researcher asks patients why *they* did not talk, or why they think they were not spoken to, and is told 'they're really sensitive those nurses — they really know when we want to be left alone'?

The point here is that collecting data about who talks to whom, and what they say, obscures the meaning of the interactions for all concerned. The same behaviour may mean different things for different people at different times. An empiricist approach to IPS can rarely take the *meaning* of the interpersonal behaviour into account; this is generally *assumed* by the researcher.

The use of empiricist approaches encourages a misunderstanding about the status of 'facts' about social behaviour. Gergen (1973) has incisively illustrated that few, if any, 'facts' about social behaviour hold true, over time. He demonstrates that the understanding and explanation of social behaviour changes with the prevailing social climate, and, furthermore, that the dissemination of the findings themselves may influence subsequent behaviour. A good illustration of this is to be found in Perrin and Spencer's (1981) attempt to replicate Asch's (1956) classical conformity study. Asch found that, in small groups, people would conform to a 'group opinion' they knew to be untrue. In 1981, Perrin found that, whilst people found it difficult to disagree with the group, they nevertheless did so. Maybe the social climate has changed between 1956 and 1981, and people nowadays are expected to conform less, and therefore do so; or maybe the 'fact' that people conform, against their better judgement, in small groups, has become so well known that people now behave differently. It would be interesting to know, for example, the extent to which TV, radio, and press coverage of ethical issues in health care (many of which focus on communication issues) and patients' rights; the increased availability of information about health and illness in the mass media, popular books and women's magazines; and the campaigns run by the Health Education Council, have changed the ways that patients behave in hospital and relate to nurses and other health professionals. If patient behaviour changes, so will the behaviour of the health professionals. Similarly, how have nurses responded to the research and documentary findings? Some of the evidence presented elsewhere in this book seems to indicate that these factors have had little effect. Nevertheless, the research is unable to illuminate the *meaning* of the findings. Do patients saying they would like more information from, or communication with nurses in 1961 (McGhee, 1961), 1978 (Reynolds, 1978) and 1984 (Forgan-Morle, 1984) all *mean* the same thing?

Given the likelihood that the explanation of social behaviour changes with situation (Argyle and Little, 1972; Argyle, Furnham and Graham, 1982) and over time, it is interesting to note that two recent 'texts', French (1983) and Smith and Bass (1982) cite about 20 per cent of references earlier than 1960. See if this book fares any better! Just as there may be problems in generalising findings from research carried out in different decades, so there may be (perhaps more obvious) problems in generalising from, say the USA to the UK. This will be particularly true of social behaviour in a professional context that differs in terms of policy, administration, organisation and practice from the one in which the research was initially conducted. Again, with reference to the two texts, over half of French's (1983) references are to foreign publications, and the bulk of Smith and Bass' (1982) are from the USA, which is not surprising, given its origins there. Davis (1981b) does draw a distinction, in his review of social skills in nursing, between work carried out in the UK and in the USA, but notes that there is little British work to draw on. This is, without doubt, changing.

Many of the so-called facts about social behaviour used to inform the IPS in nursing work are derived from laboratory experiments in social psychology. There are attendant problems with what Friedman and DiMatteo (1982) suggest is an excessively generalised application of social science matters to health issues. Newstead (1979) found that, on surveying psychology journals, 81 per cent of non-clinical studies used students as 'subjects'. Frequently they would participate in the study as part of a course requirement. Whilst there may well be a moral here for the editors of psychology journals, the nursing researcher must also beware of basing a review on the evidence of such studies. Felson (1981) demonstrated that laboratory findings did not extrapolate to real life settings, and indeed, it is important that researchers seriously consider the difficulties of generalising from one setting to another with any form of applied research.

In summary, 'facts' about social behaviour are not true for all times and all places, and furthermore, the meaning of social behaviour cannot be assumed. If the participants in the research are to contribute to meaningful research findings, then it may be necessary to adopt a humanistic approach to human nature. This may, in turn, lead to the adoption of non-empiricist forms of research.

The Validity of Research Findings

As we have seen above, and as noted by Faulkner (1984), very many research studies into IPS in nursing have been descriptive; there is, however, a move towards experimental approaches. Experimental studies invariably involve the isolation, manipulation and control of variables, and the examination of the effects on others of changing some variables. All 'irrelevant' variables are kept constant, or controlled. Within this paradigm, there are many sources of bias and distortion that can occur when the approach is adopted in the study of interpersonal behaviour. Most of the distortions occur as a result of the 'subjects' in the study attempting to gain some control over the research process, and are summarised in Table 3.1. These kinds of biases make the 'objective' and 'value free' emphasis of scientific experiments into social behaviour questionable. Take, for example, the situation of a nurse researcher conducting a study into effective communications in an antenatal clinic for her/his PhD. The nurses in the clinic either

(1) know what the research is for and what the investigation is about: they like the researcher and assume s/he is doing the research in the clinic because of its reputation for being friendly and cooperative; or

(2) have no idea who the researcher is or why s/he is doing whatever it is that s/he is doing: they are highly suspicious that 'management' is conducting a study into the efficiency of the clinic.

Table 3.1: Sources of Bias and Distortion in
Experimental Approaches to Social Behaviour

	(see e.g. Tajfel and Fraser (1978) for a discussion of these biases)
Sources in the 'Subject'	
Demand Characteristics:	Subjects have their own hypotheses about purpose of the study; they try to help or hinder the researcher.
Acquiescence	Subjects have a tendency to agree with whatever is suggested to or asked of them.
Reactance	Subjects react against the requests of the researcher
Individual Differences:	Particular characteristics will not be normally distributed amongst the population, and may therefore be difficult to take into account.
Self consciousness	Subjects may be embarrassed at being studied, and thus behave differently.
Need for approval	Subjects may want very much to be liked and thus go out of their way to be helpful.
Need for achievement	Some subjects may have a desire to do as well as they can, and even better than others.
Halo effect	Subjects may believe they have been specially chosen for the study, which may make them behave differently. Changes in certain behaviours may lead to (unexpected) changes in others.
Sources in the 'Experimenter'	
Experimenter Bias:	If the experimenters know the purpose of the study they may distort their instructions to the subjects ,or be selective in the data they collect.
Experimenter Effect:	Characteristics of the experimenters may be more or less appealing to subjects, e.g. if they are liked/disliked ;higher/equal status; male/female etc.

Will the behaviour of the nurses in the clinic be different in the two instances? One way that these pitfalls can be overcome is for the research to be unobtrusive and for the 'subjects' to know nothing about it. This, however, raises ethical problems which must be considered.

Another way, is for the 'subjects' to be fully involved in the entire research process. Reason and Rowan (1981) provide examples of several different ways of conducting participative research, all of which adopt a humanistic view of human (and social) nature.

Suitable Research into Interpersonal Skills in Nursing

It is no easy matter, in practice, to involve clinical nurses fully in research activities. Rank *et al.* (1984) offer some suggestions as to how research could be made of more practical value, and thus stand a better chance of its findings being implemented. Their recommendations are made on the assumption that 'nurse researchers', with advanced research training are available. One possibility they put forward would be for the ward sister to 'call in' a research nurse as and when a 'problem' arose for investigation; another is that the researchers could be more accountable to practising nurses than they are at present, and have a greater — and more formal — responsibility for disseminating findings directly to them; finally, the researchers themselves could be more actively involved with the delivery of care, that is, be practising nurses. None of these alternatives addresses the issue of full participation in the research process, although they do imply partial participation. Greenwood (1984) is more definite that nurse researchers studying nurse behaviour should themselves be clinical nurses. The reason for this view is that subjects and researchers should share the concepts and understanding relevant to a specific situation, if the *meaning* of behaviour that occurs is to be understood. This extreme view may be rather inhibiting — consider the implications for a researcher wishing, in part, to study the behaviour of patients! Greenwood is, though, essentially putting the case for a humanistic and phenomenological approach to nursing, claiming that nursing is:

> . . . about people, their actions and interactions, and as such is a social phenomenon . . . It is erroneous to attempt to understand any part of social reality without taking into account the way it is related to everything else . . . Any isolated nursing act is meaningless: to be understood it needs to be seen in its social context. (Greenwood, 1984, p.78)

To undertake empiricist research into IPS in nursing is to misconceive the nature of nursing, which, unlike academic social science, is a practical not a theoretical activity. In contrast to empiricist methods, Greenwood advocates action research methods that take the practical nature of nursing into account. In the light of the arguments put forward in this chapter, there are several advantages to adopting such an approach. Not only does an action research approach confine itself to diagnosing a problem in a specific context (thereby overcoming the difficulties of generalising or extrapolating from other settings), but it is also fully collaborative and participative (thereby overcoming some of the pitfalls of treating 'subjects' as 'objects'). Furthermore, it is self-evaluative, in that modifications are made continuously throughout the research process (thereby dealing in part with the issue of who defines what outcomes are acceptable). Findings might therefore stand a better chance of being seen to be relevant by the participants.

It certainly seems that, despite contention over the reliability and validity of action research, it is an approach that is particularly suited to nursing. Attempts to change some of the social aspects of nursing practice (such as the effective use of IPS) might lend themselves especially well to these methods, and indeed there are some influential precedents (e.g. Revans, 1964, 1972).

The Need for Research into Interpersonal Skills in Nursing

In the preceding discussion we have examined the nature of interpersonal skills in nursing, and critically evaluated the prevailing research paradigm. We drew attention to the possibilities for change and development of IPS, and to the specific features of the nursing context that distinguish it from other interaction contexts. We have outlined some of the difficulties of establishing criteria for desirable outcomes of the effective use of IPS in the absence of taking into account the meaning of the behaviours for all the participants. Consequently, we have argued that to adopt a more humanistic approach to the nature of people and social processes would appear to be an advance. In the light of this, we have looked at some of the shortcomings of empiricist research methods for a humanistic approach.

If nurses are to implement research findings, they must perceive them to be relevant, and we have suggested that this may be achieved if more participatory research methods are employed. There has been a great deal of research on communication in nursing — including IPS — in recent years, and yet it still appears that little change in practice has occurred (Macleod Clark, 1984). *It is now time to start engaging in*

research that will effect these changes, but to do so without the full participation of all concerned — both directly and indirectly — will be
counterproductive.

If we believe that patients will benefit from more effective use of IPS
by nurses, we must seriously consider whether or not we are entitled to
adopt controlled experimental designs that may deprive some patients
of precisely that aspect of nursing care that we have judged to be beneficial. It may well be that action research studies will prove to be the most
constructive, and least ethically dubious, way forward.

We would urge that research continue: but not just *any* research.
Instead, we would advocate that future research into IPS in nursing
adopts a humanistic view of the participants and fully involves them in
the research process; that it tries to address the question of the meaning
of interpersonal behaviours for all concerned; that it examines the
whole interaction context in which the skills are deployed; and that it
takes note of the special features of the context(s) in which practical
nursing takes place. In this way, we believe, any changes that are
induced in individuals or interpersonal systems will be more likely
to be maintained.

Note

In using the term *empiricist*, we wish to avoid confusion with *empirical methods* : at
no point do we wish to imply that observations should not be made or data collected.

References

Altschul, A. (1983) 'The Consumer's Voice: Nursing implications', *Journal of Advan-
ced Nursing, 8*, 175-83
Argyle, M. (1969) *Social Interaction*, Methuen: London
Argyle, M. (1982) *The Psychology of Interpersonal Behaviour*, Penguin: Harmonds-
worth
Argyle, M. and Kendon, A. (1967) 'The Experimental Analysis of Social Performance'
in L. Berkowitz (ed.), *Advances in Experimental Social Psychology, 3*, Academic
Press : New York
Argyle, M. and Little, B.L. (1972) 'Do Personality Traits Apply to Social Behaviour?',
Journal of the Theory of Social Behaviour, 2, 1-35
Argyle, M., Furnham, A. and Graham, J.A. (1982) *Social Situations*, Cambridge
University Press, Cambridge
Armistead, N. (1974) *Reconstructing Social Psychology*, Penguin: Harmondsworth
Asch, S.E. (1956) 'Studies of Independence and Conformity: A minority of one against
an unanimous majority', *Psychological Monographs, 70* (a) (whole no. 416)
Barton, R. (1976) *Institutional Neurosis*, Wright: Bristol (3rd edn)

Bond, S. and Bond, S. (1982) 'A Delphi Survey of Clinical Nursing Research Priorities', *Journal of Advanced Nursing*, 7, 565-75

Bridge, W. and Macleod Clark, J. (1981) *Communication in Nursing Care*, HM and M: Aylesbury

Briggs, A. (1972) *Report on the Committee of Nursing*, HMSO: London

Carkhuff, R.R. (1969) *Helping and Human Relations: A primer for lay helpers, Vols 1 & 2*, Holt, Rinehart and Winston: New York

Clark, J.M. and Hockey, L. (1979) *Research for Nursing: A guide for the enquiring nurse*, HM and M: Aylesbury

Clarke, M. (1984) 'Stress and Coping: Constructs for Nursing', *Journal of Advanced Nursing', 9*, 3-13

Crow, R. (1982) 'How Nursing and the Community can Benefit from Nursing Research', *International Journal of Nursing Studies, 19*, 37-45

Davis, B.D. (1981a) 'The Training and Assessment of Social Skills in Nursing: The patient profile interview', *Nursing Times*, April 9, 649-51

Davis, B.D. (1981b) 'Social Skills in Nursing' in M. Argyle (ed.), *Social Skills and Health*, Methuen: London

Davis, B.D. (1982) 'Social Skills Training', *Nursing Times*, October 20, 1765-8

Ellis, R.A.F. and Whittington, D. (1981) *A Guide to Social Skill Training*, Croom Helm: London

Faulkner, A. (1981) 'The Communicator as a Person', *Nursing, 27*, 1162-3

Faulkner A. (ed.) (1984) *Recent Advances in Nursing, 7, Communication* Churchill Livingstone: Edinburgh

Faulkner, A. and Maguire P. (1984) 'Teaching Assessment Skills' in A. Faulkner (ed.), *Recent Advances in Nursing, 7, Communication*, Churchill Livingstone: Edinburgh

Felson, R.B. (1981) 'Physical Attractiveness and Perceptions of Deviance', *Journal of Social Psychology, 114*, 85-9

Field, D. (1984) '"We didn't want him to die on his own" — Nurses' Accounts of Nursing Dying Patients', *Journal of Advanced Nursing, 9*, 59-70

Forgan-Morle, K.M. (1984) 'Patient Satisfaction: Care of the elderly', *Journal of Advanced Nursing, 9*, 71-6

Forrest, I. and Forrest, C. (1984) 'Relating to Patients', *Nursing Focus*, February, p.9

French, P. (1983) *Social Skills for Nursing Practice*, Croom Helm: London

Friedman, H.S. and DiMatteo, M.R. (1982) *Interpersonal Issues in Health Care*, Academic Press: New York

Gergen, K. (1973) 'Social Psychology as History', *Journal of Personality and Social Psychology, 26*, 309-20

Glaser, B.G. and Strauss, A.L. (1965) *Awareness of Dying*, Aldine: Chicago

Goffman, E. (1961) *Asylums*, Penguin: Harmondsworth (1976)

Greenwood, J. (1984) 'Nursing Research: A position paper', *Journal of Advanced Nursing, 9*, 77-82

Harré, R. and Secord, P. (1972) *The Explanation of Social Behaviour*, Blackwell: Oxford

Hitch, P.J. and Murgatroyd, J.D. (1983) 'Professional Communications in Cancer Care: A Delphi study of hospital nurses', *Journal of Advanced Nursing, 8*, 413-22

Hunt, J. (1984) 'Why Don't We Use These Findings?' *Nursing Mirror*, 22 February, p.29

Israel, J. and Tajfel, H. (eds) (1972) *The Context of Social Psychology: A Critical Assessment*, Academic Press: London

Kagan, C. and Burton, M. (1982) 'Scenes of Improvement', *Nursing Mirror*, 18 August, 44-5

Kagan, N. (1975) 'Influencing Human Interaction — Eleven years with IPR', *Canadian Counsellor, 9*, 74-97

Kelly, M.P. and May, D. (1982) 'Good and Bad Patients: A review of the literature and a theoretical critique', *Journal of Advanced Nursing*, 7, 147-56

Knight, M. and Field, D. (1981) 'A Silent Conspiracy: Coping with dying cancer patients on an acute surgical ward', *Journal of Advanced Nursing*, 6, 221-9

Macleod Clark, J. (1981a) 'Communication in Nursing', *Nursing Times*, January 1, 12-18

Macleod Clark, J. (1981b) 'Communications with Cancer Patients: Communication or evasion?' in R. Tiffany (ed.), *Cancer Nursing Update*, Balliere Tindall: London

Macleod Clark, J. (1983) 'Nurse-Patient Communication: An analysis of conversations from surgical wards' in J. Wilson Barnett (ed.), *Nursing Research: Ten studies in patient care*, Wiley: Chichester

Macleod Clark, J. (1984) 'Verbal Communication in Nursing' in A. Faulkner (ed.), *Recent Advances in Nursing*, 7, *Communication*, Churchill Livingstone: Edinburgh

McGhee, A. (1961) *The Patients' Attitude to Nursing Care*, E. and S.L. Livingstone: Edinburgh

McIntee, J. and Firth, H. (1984) 'How To Beat the Burnout', *Health and Social Services Journal*, February 9, 166-8

McIntosh, J. (1977) *Communication and Awareness in a Cancer Ward*, Croom Helm: London

Murray, M. (1983) 'Role Conflict and Intention to Leave Nursing', *Journal of Advanced Nursing*, 8, 29-31

Newstead, S.E. (1979) 'Student Subjects in Psychological Experiment', *Bulletin of the British Psychological Society*, 32, 384-6

Orford, J. (1981) 'Institutional Climates' in J.D. Hall (ed.), *Psychology for Nurses and Health Visitors*, Macmillan: London

Parsons, T. (1951) *The Social System*, Routledge and Kegan Paul: London

Perrin, S. and Spencer, C. (1981) 'Independence or Conformity in the Asch Experiment as a Reflection of Cultural and Situational Factors', *British Journal of Social Psychology*, 20, 205-9

Rabkin, J.G. and Struening, E.L. (1976) 'Life Events, Stress and Illness', Science, 194, 1013-20

Rank, P., Rostron, W. and Stenhouse, M. (1984) 'Using Research in Nursing', *Nursing Times*, March 14, 44-5

Reason, P. and Rowan, J. (1981) *Human Enquiry: A sourcebook of new paradigm research*, Wiley: Chichester

Revans, R.W. (1964) *Standards for Morale: Cause and effect in hospitals*, Oxford University Press: London

Revans, R.W. (1972) *Hospitals and Communication, Choice and Change*, Tavistock: London

Reynolds, M. (1978), 'No News is Bad News: Patients' views about communication in hospital', *British Medical Journal*, 1, 1673-6

Roberts, D. (1984) 'Non-Verbal Communication: Popular and unpopular patients', in A. Faulkner (Ed.), *Recent Advances in Nursing*, 7: *Communication*, Churchill Livingstone: Edinburgh

Rosenhan, D.L. (1973) 'On Being Sane in Insane Places', *Science*, 179, 250-8

Royal College of Nursing in the United Kingdom (1978) *Counselling in Nursing*, RCN: London

Smith, V.M. and Bass, T.A. (1982) *Communication for the Health Care Team* (adapted by A. Faulkner) Harper and Row: London

Stockwell, F. (1972) *The Unpopular Patient*, RCN: London (Republished by Croom Helm, London, 1984)

Tajfel, H. and Fraser, C. (1978) *Introducing Social Psychology*, Penguin: Harmondsworth

Wolpe, J. (1969) *The Practice of Behavior Therapy*, Aldine: Chicago

PART II:

THE CONTEXT OF INTERPERSONAL SKILLS IN NURSING

Nursing as we have seen, takes place in an interaction context: the individual skills of nurses are partly determined by that context. However, the organisational, environmental and wider social/political contexts in which nursing takes place also influence the effective use of interpersonal skills.

Ann Faulkner, in *Chapter 4*, considers how the nursing curricula, the attitudes and priorities of managers, and the imbalance of the doctor-nurse relationship are all organisational obstacles to the effective deployment of interpersonal skills. Furthermore, she notes that the organisation of ward work is more often 'task' allocated, rather than 'individual patient care' allocated. Faulkner is optimistic that moves towards greater 'individual patient care' allocation of work will necessitate greater use of effective interpersonal skills. This might, in turn, ensure that changes to curricula are introduced, in order to prepare nurses for this different way of working. A further consequence of these changes, however, will be nurses' increased need for personal support from both management and peers, and a greater requirement for interpersonal relationships *between* professionals to be examined.

A more sceptical note is introduced by *Mark Burton* in *Chapter 5*. He argues that the expected effects of more humanistic and individualised patient care, once the nursing process is brought into effect, may not occur, owing to the particular features of the environment into which it is to be introduced. The hospital is, he suggests, a strange place where strange things happen to people. There is no analogue in the ordinary world, and by entering it, we leave familiar environments where our interpersonal skills work for an unfamiliar environment where they have lost many of their setting events. Burton presents the health service culture as one that focuses on the physical definition of needs, professional role distance and those special features that make the environment such a strange place. As such, he maintains that hospitals present a 'triumph of deculturation', wherein the opportunities for interaction are too few and tend to be too brief, and wherein several forces — both structural and ideological — work against their having appropriate content. If changes are to be brought about in the effective use of interpersonal skills by nurses, he asserts, it will not just be by concentrating on the training of individual nurses: rather, changes in the environments and culture of health care, and in the medical definition of health, are called for.

Perhaps the most challenging note of all is struck by *Francis Lillie*, who, in *Chapter 6*, discusses the wider social context of nursing. This is characterised by political and moral issues that effect the morale of those working in, and using the health services. The development of health systems is seen to be the result of political pressures external to the needs of the populations they serve. This makes individual responses to patients' needs by nurses difficult to achieve. For nurses to understand this fully, he argues, they should be aware of methods of health care funding and problematic aspects of the National Health Service system. He singles out for special attention the medical domination of the NHS; the language that communicates images to the health workers and their patients; the secrecy surrounding NHS policy making; and the problems of access to health advice and care for priority groups. Part II ends on an optimistic note, though, as Lillie advocates the merger of personal and professional selves, and calls upon all of us to challenge the social/political/economic status of our work.

4 THE ORGANISATIONAL CONTEXT OF INTERPERSONAL SKILLS IN NURSING

Ann Faulkner

Introduction

Nursing as a profession has a hierarchical structure in which managers, from ward sister upwards, make decisions about the organisation of patient care, and the priorities of that care. They do not, of course, work in isolation but in collaboration with other members of the health care team, some of whom are seen to impose their own priorities in terms of patient care. Nurses learn their skills in both the classroom and the ward. They will learn to put a value on interpersonal skills only if such skills are taught in the school *and* observed in the ward as a priority within the organisation of health care. There is a considerable research literature to suggest that in the area of communication nurses have considerable deficiencies (e.g. Ashworth, 1980; Faulkner, 1980; Macleod Clark, 1982; Maguire, Tait and Brook, 1980). Peter Maguire (Chapter 8) considers these deficiencies. This present chapter is concerned with the organisational factors which may affect nurses' ability to develop their interpersonal skills both in terms of the organisation of the curricula and the nurses' ward experience.

The Curricula

Until recently, nursing has been organised on what is popularly called the 'medical model'. This means that emphasis has been placed on learning about disease and its treatment. As a result, physiology has had an important place in curricula and blocks of study have concentrated on specialities such as 'medicine', 'surgery', and 'care of the elderly'. It is easy in a system of this sort for nurses to feel that they are looking after conditions rather than individuals.

A newer approach to nursing is that of the 'nursing process' (e.g. Kratz, 1980; McFarlane and Castledine, 1982) in which a move has been made towards more individualised care. The process is usually divided into four stages of assessment, planning, implementation and evaluation, and the approach is one of problem-solving on an individual basis. The GNC syllabus of nursing (1977) suggests that the nursing process should be used in nursing care. This should have resulted in curriculum changes to reflect new thinking. However, nurse tutors on study days often comment that lectures are given on the nursing process but that they are separate from other teaching on nursing. If this is so, then it is reasonable to suppose that curricula in many schools may still be organised on a medical model, which militates against the teaching of interpersonal skills.

Interpersonal Skills and the Process of Nursing

The process approach to nursing should rely heavily on interpersonal skills particularly in assessment which is seen as a dynamic, ongoing part of care. Faulkner (1981) suggests that without the appropriate interactive skills, care may be planned on insufficient information and may not be appropriate to the individual patient. Of the three-years training period for registered general nurses (RGN), 26 weeks are spent in the school. If most of this is still tied to the medical approach to nursing it can be seen that there may be difficulties in adding material such as interpersonal skills to curricula without taking something out, or extending the theoretical part of training. In order to assess patients' problems, nurses need the skills of interviewing as well as basic interpersonal skills with which to approach patients and make them feel comfortable, so that they will disclose their problems.

To obtain some data on the place of communication skills in curricula, and attitudes towards teaching this subject which is so crucial to the nursing process, a survey was carried out of all Directors of Nurse Education (DNE) in England, Wales and Northern Ireland (Faulkner, Bridge and Macleod Clark, 1983). The high response rate to this survey (84 per cent) suggests that DNEs are concerned with the place of interpersonal skills in curricula. However, in response to the question 'At a rough guess, what percentage of time is spent on planned communication sessions in SRN training?', 32.4 per cent responded that 5 per cent or less time was given, while 43.4 per cent thought that less than 10 per cent of time was given to the subject. Added to this was the opinion that only 10.3 per cent of tutors are well prepared to teach communication skills and only 2.1 per cent very well prepared. It may be assumed from this report that the small amount of time which is spent on teaching interactive skills may be of little use if tutors have not had the preparation for teaching the subject. Hussey (1981), when studying the teaching of communication skills in one school of nursing, found that some teachers were uncomfortable with experiential teaching methods and that others did not themselves appear to have effective communication skills.

While the move towards using a nursing process approach to care is limited to a few disconnected lectures, it seems unlikely that it can be seen as a vehicle for a change in emphasis towards developing interpersonal skills in nursing. A reorganisation of curricula appears to be required which emphasises the patient as an individual, and which has interactive skills as a core subject which feeds into all other aspects of care. This does not mean that nurses will no longer be interested in medical diagnosis, for they could not nurse safely without such knowledge. It does mean, though, that diagnosis will be seen more in terms of its effects on an individual than has been possible in the medical model of nursing. Basic training is not the only place where interpersonal skills may be learned, but no matter what other training is undertaken, e.g. District Nursing, Health Visiting or Midwifery, most ask for basic RGN registration as a prerequisite to training. It is, therefore, vital that the basic curricula should be organised to equip nurses with appropriate interpersonal skills so that post-basic courses may build on a firm foundation when teaching more sophisticated skills such as counselling. In research which is currently being undertaken, and which is funded by the Health Education Council (HEC), an experimental programme of interpersonal skills is being taught in selected schools of nursing during the first fifteen months of basic nurse training. Evaluation of the programme may well show that curricula need to be reorganised to include both planned sessions on interactive skills and consolidation sessions where skills learned can be interwoven with particular aspects of nursing care.

Interpersonal Skills on the Ward

In Faulkner *et al.*'s (1983) study, 32 per cent of DNEs thought the ward was the most appropriate place for nurses to learn to communicate with patients. In spite of this, it is not uncommon for nurses to return to the school after their first ward experience and say 'As soon as I tried to talk to patients, someone would ask me to do something else'. Student nurses soon learn that interacting with patients is seen as a waste of time. This is borne out by research in which nurse-patient conversations were recorded (Faulkner, 1980; Macleod Clark, 1982) and found to be very short and usually linked with performing a task on, or for, the patients.

Traditionally, wards have been organised on the basis of task allocation. This means that nurses are assigned tasks for a span of duty such as 'observation', 'fluid balance', 'bedbaths' or 'drugs'. Organising a ward in this way may be seen to be effective in terms of staff time, but it does tend to fragment care and reduce interaction. Faulkner (1980), on observing nurse-patient interaction on a ward, found that it was possible and quite common for a nurse to approach a patient, carry out a task, e.g. TPR or inhalation, and walk away without any verbal exchange occurring. The aim of the nursing process is that care will be given on the basis of 'patient' rather than 'task' allocation. Ideally, a nurse, or nurses, will give total patient care to a few patients for the length of their stay in hospital. This change in organisation of the ward should mean that nurses will be able to build relationships with their patients. For this they will need improved interactive skills and encouragement to use them.

Trained Staff as Role Models

If the ward is an appropriate place for nurses to learn to develop interpersonal skills, the question arises as to how this learning should take place. Clinical teachers may come to the ward to teach learners, but personal experience of assessing clinical teachers suggests that most teaching is geared to nursing tasks, e.g. bedbathing, drug rounds, the giving of injections and the care of pressure areas. If the nurse learns interpersonal skills it will be because of the effect of role modelling.

Lelean (1973), in studying the organisation of the ward sister's communication on the ward, found that only 2 per cent of the sister's time was spent in interacting with first year students. This suggests that as a role model the ward sister is elusive. Other trained staff, including the clinical teacher and staff nurse, may spend more time with the learners although it is not unusual to find quite junior nurses working together, nor to hear a learner comment 'I might do better in my assessments if a clinical teacher were to come and help me'. If the ideal situation occurred where learners were exposed to trained staff as role models, would interpersonal skills improve? Faulkner and Maguire (1984) found that trained nurses on a surgical ward had many deficiencies in interpersonal skills but did not recognise that they had such deficiencies. It can be assumed that trained nurses such as these will not be able to teach learners interpersonal skills, since they do not themselves possess them. Any role modelling will be in a negative direction and each new generation of nurses will continue the poor pattern of communication suggested by current research.

Faulkner and Maguire's (1984) study included the training of trained ward staff on their own ward. These nurses were asked to tape record assessment interviews with mastectomy patients and were shown how to improve on their performance by positive feedback. Interpersonal skills improved dramatically in a short time. After the study was completed, ward routine was reorganised to include not only assessment of all patients, but teaching of all student nurses who gain experience on that ward. Although this part of the study concentrated on one ward and eight nurses, it could be tentatively suggested that, with appropriate training, ward sisters and staff nurses could act as role models for learners in the area of interpersonal skills. However, Faulkner and Maguire did find problems both in motivating staff and in gaining the co-operation of management.

If the ward is to be accepted as an appropriate place for learners to develop interpersonal skills, trained staff need to be willing to learn those skills which were absent in their own training and to reorganise the ward towards the process approach to give more emphasis to meaningful interaction with patients. Management needs to be co-operative because the changes envisaged are quite radical. The traditional idea that all the routine ward work will be completed by 11.00 a.m. may need to change and priorities may have to be revised. The Sister may be more prepared to do this if the Nursing Officer is interested and supportive. Other members of the health care team also need to be understanding and supportive if the ward is to be reorganised to improve patient care. It is particularly important to gain the co-operation of medical staff whose roles are closely interrelated with those of nurses. The medical model of nursing tended to throw nurses into a subservient, 'personal assistant' role to the doctor and this image, if it lingers, may hamper nurses in their interactions with patients.

The Medical Influence

The medical influence on ward organisation and therefore on patterns of communication cannot be ignored. This is particularly true in the area of information-giving to both patients and relatives. As one ward sister put it, when on a study day on communication, 'It's all right for you to talk of improving communication with patients. You should meet my consultant — he won't let me tell the patients a bloody thing!'. If consultants are controlling nurses in this way one must ask why such control should occur and why nursing staff should accept it. It may be that the consultant feels responsible to the point of dictating policy, but it may also be because of poor communication between nurse and doctor so that the implications of control are not properly understood.

Doctors and nurses are colleagues, united in their common aim towards improved patient care. Their roles are interdependent and as such should be cooperative. It is only the hang-ups from the 'personal assistant' image that throw the doctor into the role of tyrant, for as Gilbran (1979) asks, 'How can a tyrant rule the free and the proud, but for a tyranny in their own freedom and a shame in their own pride?' If medical staff do control information to patients, this can cause problems for nurses in their interactive roles. Nothing is more inhibiting to interpersonal exchange than a secret, and the more important the secret, the more inhibiting it is to easy interaction. In nursing, the area where nurses feel most inhibited by medical opinion appears to be in fear-provoking diagnosis or prognosis.

Because nurses do not generally accept that their relationship with the medical profession is one of colleagues in the organisational context of nursing care, there is still an implicit belief that doctors can dictate what a patient may or may not be told. Too often the decision is based on the personal beliefs of the individual doctor rather than on an assessment of each individual patient. Such a situation may cause difficulties for the nurse who has assessed the patient's needs to be different from those dictated by the doctor. It is probably true to say that nowhere is this more apparent than when a patient has an irreversible disease or is terminally ill.

There is an enormous literature on the subject of 'to tell or not to tell' patients the truth if they are dying, yet if nursing is organised on a nursing process approach such a fraught question need not exist. If a nurse assesses a patient's needs for knowledge and meets those needs, some patients will be told the truth while others may continue to deny the real state of affairs and may die without discussion. The importance of patients receiving only that information for which they are ready needs to be understood by all health professionals, and for this to happen the skills of perception and assessment are of paramount importance. Many nurses feel constrained by the organisational expectations in this area and fear that meeting the patient's expressed needs may offend a consultant who has asked that diagnosis be kept from an individual. This situation may only change if nurses are prepared to have faith and accept responsibility for those decisions. Doctors can only respect nurses who have the courage of their convictions, particularly since the result can be patients who, after the initial upset of bad news, are usually more settled once they can make sense of what is occurring to them.

The relationship between doctors and nurses needs further exploration if the organisation of patient care is to improve, especially in the area of interpersonal skills. Personal experience has shown that nurses often feel unable to interact comfortably with a patient because they are unaware of medical policy and feel that it is inappropriate to show ignorance before a patient. This situation again shows the need for nurses to develop effective interpersonal skills, for it is possible to ask a patient 'What do you understand about your illness?' without appearing ignorant. Further, it should be possible for nurses to take part in a dialogue with doctors so that joint decisions may be made on meeting patients' needs for communication.

Since the need to improve interpersonal skills appears to be common to all nurses, consideration needs to be given to in-service training, for if Faulkner and Maguire's (1984) study is an indication of what can be achieved, it is reasonable to suppose that concentrating efforts on trained nurses will also help improve the skills of learners both through role models and active teaching on the ward.

In-service Teaching of Interpersonal Skills

The major organisational constraint to teaching interpersonal skills to trained nurses through in-service training is the conflict between service needs from the nurses and the nurses' need for further education. A strong case may be made that if nurses can update their knowledge through continuing education then patient care will improve. However, the other side of the coin is that of the immediate needs of the patients. Few managers feel able to risk low levels of staff on the wards today for improved care tomorrow. Since it is not mandatory for clinical nurses to take refresher courses (with the exception of midwives) it can be seen that in-service education may have a low priority for nurses and managers alike. On a more optimistic note, hospitals normally do have an in-service training officer and a budget for further education so the possibility does exist for nurses to update skills or learn new ones.

In-service training may take the form of study days or short courses of one or two weeks. More emphasis is being given on these courses to interpersonal skills, both at the basic interactive level and at the more sophisticated level of counselling and interaction with the bereaved. As with basic learners, however, unless the organisation of nursing care allows for these skills to be used, the gap between theory and practice will continue and patient care will not improve. When the organisational structure allows time for up-dating of nurses' skills, often too much is expected in terms of what can be achieved in a short time. Faulkner and Maguire (1984) point out that short workshops can be expected to do no more than raise awareness of the problems of meaningful interaction with patients, both in what it demands of nurses and of the skills required. Nevertheless, if workshops do raise awareness, the first steps are being taken to improve interpersonal skills.

Interpersonal Skills in the Community

Nurses who wish to work in the community as district nurses or health visitors are required to undertake a course before they are judged competent to practise. Traditionally, the district nurse has been seen as essentially a practical nurse while the health visitor's role has been seen as largely preventative. It could be argued from this that the course for health visitors as outlined by the Council for the Education and Training of Health Visitors (1981) would rely heavily on the teaching of interpersonal skills, whereas district nurses' courses would give more emphasis to practical skills. Current research on the aftercare of mastectomy patients appears to suggest that in spite of differently organised courses there is little to choose between the interpersonal skills of district nurses and health visitors. Indeed the emerging picture is of the same deficiencies as are found in general nurses. As one health visitor commented 'We are not taught these (interpersonal) skills so that we are able to counsel. All we are taught is to guide and advise'.

Another factor which affects nurses' attitudes to interpersonal skills in the community is the influence of management, both in terms of priorities in the communities and expectations of the role of health visitors and district nurses. Turton and Faulkner (1983) suggest that district nursing management are more impressed with figures of injections given and bedbaths performed than with observational visits to patients with emotional problems. Of course one can argue that these nurses may well interact effectively with those patients with whom they come into contact, although Kratz (1978) suggests that district nurses do not have the communication skills required to assess their patients.

Community care is organised in such a way that the General Practitioner (GP) is seen as head of the health care team. This may mean that community nurses are meeting two sets of demands (i.e. those of the nursing manager and of the GP). If GPs do not believe that district nurses should give psychosocial care, they may not refer any patients except those who need physical care. Although district nurses may initiate visits, they do need to know which patients need their help. Most referrals come from the GP. Others may come direct from the hospital but here the usual cause of referral is that the patient needs physical care.

Health visitors may be seen to be in a happier position to give psychological care for which interpersonal skills are so essential, since they carry their own case loads. Here again, though, there are organisational constraints, not least in the perception of priorities. In current research, three district managers refused access to health visitors because their priorities are seen to be the 0-5 age group and the project involved adults.

Although organisational factors cannot prevent nurses from developing their interpersonal skills, they can have an influence in terms of priorities. If district nurse managers do not see the importance of meaningful interaction with patients, they are more likely to reward evidence of physical rather than emotional care. In these circumstances it is a brave nurse who reduces the number of bedbaths in favour of observational visits. Similarly with health visitors. If the 0-5 age group are seen as priorities, those clients outside this range are unlikely to be given much attention. This means that many patients who are known to develop psychological problems after discharge, e.g. mastectomy, hysterectomy and cancer patients, may be neglected simply because they do not fall into the recognised net of either district nurse or health visitor.

Acceptance of the need for development and use of interpersonal skills by nursing management in the community could well affect the case loads of both district nurses and health visitors. The problem of staffing levels may well be a factor in current decision making, but ignoring the problems caused by poor or no assessment could well be costing money in psychiatric care.

Conclusions

There seems little doubt from research findings that nurses both in hospital and community settings have severe deficiencies in interpersonal skills. Some of these deficiencies may be seen to be due to deficits in the curricula — of both basic and post-basic courses — and in a reluctance or inability on the part of tutors to use experiential methods of teaching. Other organisational factors which inhibit nurses from developing interpersonal skills may be seen to be the attitudes and priorities of managers and the imbalance of the relationship between doctors and nurses, this latter causing nurses to say 'nothing' rather than to say the wrong thing to a patient. The actual organisation of ward work has also been shown to affect interaction with patients if it is organised on a task allocation basis and it may be here that the clue to improvement will be found.

Reorganisation of nursing care on an individualised basis makes explicit the need for nurses at all levels to develop interpersonal skills. Since change more often comes from need than good ideas, the future may see increasing emphasis on interpersonal skills. When that occurs, curricula may change. Current research, such as the HEC-funded project in basic nurse training and the project described by Faulkner and Maguire (1984), suggests that interpersonal skills can be taught, the latter project suggesting that skills learnt can be maintained over time in the right atmosphere and with support.

The notion of support is crucial, for if interpersonal skills are used by nurses for a better understanding of their patients, the defence mechanisms described by Jourard (1964) and Menzies (1970) will have to be abandoned. This means that nurses will come much closer to their patients' pain. Support and understanding from management and/ or preferably from a peer support group will then be necessary so that nurses may share the professional problems inherent in dealing with patients' emotional needs.

Finally, communication between health professionals must be seen as a priority in the organisation of patient care since if we do not interact with each other, patient care becomes fragmented and confused.

Acknowledgements

I would like to acknowledge other directors of the HEC-funded project 'Communication in Nurse Education' (CINE), Will Bridge, Jill Macleod Clark and Jane Randell. I would also like to acknowledge the unfailing help of Peter Maguire in the study on teaching nurses assessment skills, which is DHSS-funded.

References

Ashworth, P. (1980) *Care to Communicate*, RCN: London

Council for the Education and Training of Health Visitors (1981) *Guide to Syllabus of Training*, UKCC: London

Faulkner, A. (1980) 'The Student Nurses' Role in Giving Information to Patients', unpublished M. Litt. thesis: Aberdeen University

Faulkner, A. (1981) 'Aye, There's the Rub', *Nursing Times*, 77, 332-6

Faulkner, A., Bridge, W. and Macleod Clark, J. (1983) 'Teaching Communication in Schools of Nursing: a survey of Directors of Nurse Education', Paper given at RCN Conference: Brighton

Faulkner, A. and Maguire, P. (1984) 'Teaching Assessment Skills', in A. Faulkner (ed.), *Recent Advances in Nursing*, 7, *Communication*, Churchill Livingstone: Edinburgh

General Nursing Council for England and Wales (1977) *Training Syllabus for Register of Nurses*, GNC: London

Gilbran, K. (1979) *The Prophet*, Heinemann: London

Hussey, A. (1981) 'Interpersonal communication skills in nursing', unpublished MSc thesis: University of Aston in Birmingham

Jourard, S. (1964) *The Transparent Self*, Van Nostrand: Princetown, N.J.

Kratz, C. (1978) *Care of the Long Term Sick in the Community*, Churchill Livingstone: Edinburgh

Kratz, C. (1980) *The Nursing Process*, Bailliere Tindall: London (3rd Edn)

Lelean, S. (1973) *Ready for Report, Nurse?* RCN: London

Maguire, P., Tait, A. and Brook, M. (1980) 'A Conspiracy of Pretence', *Nursing Mirror*, 150, 17-19

Macleod Clark, J. (1982) 'Nurse-patient verbal interaction', unpublished PhD thesis: University of London

McFarlane, J. and Casteldine, G. (1982) *A Guide to the Practice of Nursing*, Mosby: London

Menzies, I. (1970) *Defence Systems as Control Against Anxiety*, Tavistock: London

Turton, P. and Faulkner, A. (1983) 'Carer and Educator', *Journal of District Nursing*, 2, 20, 22

5 THE ENVIRONMENT, GOOD INTERACTIONS AND INTERPERSONAL SKILLS IN NURSING

Mark Burton

Introduction

Interpersonal skills are not an end, but a means to an end. The end is 'good interactions' for the users of the service (patients or clients). Just what a good interaction is will depend upon the needs of the user, both at the moment a particular interaction takes place (e.g. need for relief of pain, need to express worries), and within the longer-term development of that person (e.g. need to acquire better ways of relating to other people, need to learn to feed oneself, need to review one's life history prior to dying). To happen effectively, interactions

(1) have to actually take place;
(2) have to be sustained for as long as necessary, rather than being cut off prematurely;
(3) have to have an appropriate content.

In what follows I shall assume that all three conditions could be made more likely through appropriate training, but I will argue that despite this, the way the environment is structured can do much to create these conditions, and where it is structured in a way *inimical* to these conditions, then training will be largely a waste of time, except in so far as it raises consciousness of these issues. The argument will be supported by reference to research literature, but it is actually largely a matter of simple logic.

The three conditions for good interactions, (1) initiation, (2) maintenance of contact, and (3) appropriate content, are generally met in everyday life. It is when people find themselves in unaccustomed situations (e.g. in hospital or in staff-patient role relationships) that things start going wrong. Most of us, then, get by fairly well in ordinary interactions: there is a big reservoir of skill there already, that is the common property of anyone who is a participating member of our culture. It is hard to imagine what would happen were this not so, but it would clearly be difficult to get many quite mundane things done, and we would probably spend a lot of time feeling pretty uncomfortable in each other's presence. So can the problem with nursing really be one of interpersonal skill, and can the problem be fixed through a massive injection of skills training throughout the nursing professions? As Desmond Cormack (Chapter 7) points out, psychiatric nurses actually have considerable interpersonal skills for doing certain things — how could they survive otherwise? As I shall argue, the problem with interactions in health care settings is one of 'deculturation' — the dislocation of people from the ordinary cultural settings in which they function effectively, and that in a variety of ways embody values that are seen as important in our culture, such as dignity, respect, privacy, autonomy and choice. The solution requires radical and challenging answers — the transfer of health and social care to ordinary cultural contexts wherever this is technically possible, and a relinquishing of many so called 'professional' values in the caring professions.

Opportunities for Interaction : Frequency and Duration

Good interactions, then, depend firstly on there being a chance for contact to be made between people. The physical layout of an environment can strongly influence this. Consider the following set-up:

Forty-two elderly people (nearly all women) sit by day in a windowless room. All have mental disabilities, the majority having lost some of their mental powers, while a large proportion are physically frail. There are staff, but only enough to keep pace with the demands of physical care, with the exception of two nursing assistants whose work in the afternoon is described as 'occupational therapy' (no OT or other staff give them support or guidance in this work, with the exception of a clinical psychology student getting his MSc thesis and a publication, Burton (1980), from this ward).

If you are one of the elderly people you have few opportunities for 'good interactions'. Your chances are as follows:

(1) With one another, but then your neighbour is also likely to be disorientated, or depressed, or just tired.

(2) With the nursing staff — when it's your turn for the toilet or some other bit of physical care.

(3) With the OT aide, when she is not working with one of the 41 others.

(4) With the doctor — in this case a very caring and skilled man — who does manage to visit twice a week for an hour or so.

(5) With the psychology student, or his clipboard?

(6) With visitors, ancillary staff, and anyone else who comes on to the ward.

The chances of contact don't look good for anyone here, but for some people, arguably those with the greatest need for contact with others, the chances are less than for others. Observation of this set-up in practice showed that the people who had deteriorated the most tended to sit around the walls of the room, while the rest were seated around three large tables, as follows:

Table 1. The least deteriorated people were seated on this table. The table was situated (a) near to the corridor leading to the ward office; (b) next to the small kitchen, used by the ward staff; (c) on the routes from both the back entrance of the ward, and the next-door ward, to the nursing office; (d) on the routes from the nursing office, the front entrance and the staff kitchen to the toilets; (e) next to the cupboard where OT equipment was kept; and (f) next to the telephone in the day room.

Table 2. More deteriorated residents were seated around this table. It was (a) on the route from the neighbouring ward to the rest of this ward; (b) next to the radiogram; and (c) near, but not on, the route to the back entrance to the ward.

Table 3. A similar group of people to those on Table 2, occupied this table. It was in the corner of the day room on the route to the toilets, but on no other routes.

Over two afternoon sessions, the number of visits by staff (of all types) to each of the tables was counted. A 'visit' was defined as when someone stopped at the table for five seconds or more, whether or not they interacted with the elderly people. The tables were visited at the following average frequencies per hour (corrected for number of people sitting at each table) : Table 1 : 38, Table 2 : 14, Table 3 : 18.

While we cannot be certain why those at Table 1 got more than twice the opportunities for interaction than those at either Table 2 or 3, it seems likely that the favourable position of Table 1 near to all the major routes through the room was a big factor. Whilst people on Table 1 might have been easier to chat with than the others, it is also likely that this is why they had been put in the favoured position. Similarly, Blackman, Howe and Pinkston (1976) demonstrated that elderly people in a nursing home were more likely to interact with one another when coffee was served to them in a sun-lounge than when they received it in their habitual chairs.

Zimring, Weitzer and Knight (1982) found that remodelling wards at a Massachusetts institution for people with mental handicaps led to slight increases in interactions among residents but a decrease in interactions between residents and staff. Holahan (1979) similarly reported significant changes in various measures of social interaction at a psychiatric hospital as a result of remodelling ward environments. In both cases partitions and furniture rearrangements were used to provide increased personal space. The physical layout of the environment, then, can influence whether interactions occur. So can social aspects of the setting.

It is interesting to compare some studies carried out in various hospital environments. Sanson-Fisher and Poole (1979), studied a psychiatric unit in a general hospital. Making observations of staff and client activity throughout the unit, they found staff spent 23.5 per cent of their time interacting with clients, 41 per cent interacting with other staff, 3.6 per cent with other people and 31.8 per cent in solitary activity. (Figures are given for all types of staff: nursing staff fall in the middle, between professional staff who interacted with clients less, and occupational therapists, who did so more.) As these authors point out, 'potential therapeutic opportunities are being missed'. The staff, however, believed (on average) that 62 per cent of their time should be devoted to interaction with clients. Whatever the staff's awareness of the need for interactions, some features of the environment seem to have reduced the opportunities for them.

Sanson-Fisher *et al.* (1979) were studying a unit at a University teaching hospital, but in many institutional environments the opportunity for interaction is considerably lower. We (Cullen, Burton, Watts and Thomas, 1983) studied a mental handicap hospital, and looked at two environments, a ward and a recreational day centre. We looked at the interactions experienced by ten men who were representative of the middle of the range of residents in terms of their handicaps. In the ward, 93 per cent of their time was spent not interacting, while the proportion in the recreation hall was 92 per cent. Interactions with staff lasted an average of 11.23 seconds. These findings are in line with those of Grant

(1974) who, in two mental handicap hospitals, found that 42.8 and 63 per cent (respectively) of interactions were of less than ten seconds duration, and that there was an average of 26.5 and 20.1 minutes between interactions. Finally, in a study of a long-stay psychiatric hospital, Fox (1983) found that patients in two 'long-stay/rehabilitation wards' were engaged in solitary behaviour on 78.1 per cent of the occasions they were observed throughout the day. In the latter two types of setting, staffing levels are not high, but even where they are better (as in Sanson-Fisher, 1979), the opportunities for interaction are fewer than staff themselves judge to be appropriate.

It seems that the finding of infrequent and brief interactions between nurses and clients/patients is not restricted to the 'Cinderella services'. Macleod Clark, reviewing literature from a wide variety of settings, including general surgical and medical wards, concludes that,

> It can be seen, therefore that the general pattern of one-to-one verbal communication that emerges is one of infrequent interaction, of short duration, which occurs mostly in conjunction with a specific nursing activity. (Macleod Clark, 1984, p.62)

So, in a variety of hospital settings, the opportunities for interaction with clients are few. We have seen how the physical layout of the environment can influence these opportunities (Blackman *et al.*, 1976; Burton, 1979; Holahan, 1979; Zimring *et al.*, 1982).

Other factors can play a role too. In the environments studied by us (Cullen *et al.*, 1983), by Fox (1983), and by Grant (1974), for example, staffing levels are going to be a limiting factor, although more effective use of the available staff (e.g. through a 'room management' — Porterfield, Blunden and Blewitt, 1980 — or similar scheme (Burton, 1980)) might improve matters within certain limits. However, as Sanson-Fisher *et al.* (1979) showed, even where staffing levels were high, the opportunities for interaction were fewer than staff themselves saw as desirable. They attributed this to two factors, firstly competing tasks for staff (e.g. bureaucratic tasks and meetings), and secondly, the availability of more rewarding interactions for staff members — they seemed to prefer talking to staff people than to client people.

I would also suggest that in settings where mentally disabled people are cared for, the pervasive negative view of such people in our culture is another factor. The segregation of these people from their communities (historically a major role of professionals), low expectations of their capabilities or potential (often legitimated by medical ideology), and explanations of behaviour that situate causes within the person — these influences probably lie behind the not-so-unfamiliar picture of the nurses reading the paper in their office while the people kick their heels in the day room. This all means that not only is our first condition rarely met (opportunities for interactions to be initiated), but what data we have suggest that the interactions themselves are generally very brief, thereby possibly violating our second condition (there should be a chance for contact to be maintained).

Content of Interactions

For interactions to be good ones, that is for them to have a chance of being a vehicle for meeting the needs of clients, they also have to have appropriate content. The question arises: how do we define appropriateness of content? Behavioural psychology gives us an idea for a *minimum* definition of appropriate content:

> . . . defined appropriate behaviour should be consistently responded to with positive attention, while inappropriate behaviour should be ignored or punished. (Sanson-Fisher and Poole, 1980, p.145; after Ayllon and Michael, 1959)

Clearly this is a very minimal definition of a 'good interaction', and one that only really applies to services for people with major behavioural excesses or deficits. It is a highly mechanistic definition (we might ponder on the fact that it could only be penned in a context of extreme differences between the relative power of clients and staff). It also makes an assumption about the rewarding quality of attention from nurses (an assumption, however, that is, likely to be warranted for many of the clients, much of the time, given the paucity of such environments). Nevertheless, the very *minimal* quality of this definition of appropriate content makes it interesting for us to test whether interactions in health care environments meet even this standard.

Gelfand, Gelfand and Dobson (1967) found that psychiatric nursing staff gave positive attention to clients' behaviour whether or not the behaviour was appropriate. Moreover, they found that other clients applied attention more discriminately. Sanson-Fisher and Poole (1980) divided behaviour into three categories: *appropriate* ('positive self-concept', 'independent altruism', and ordinary conversation); *neutral* (on-task behaviour); and *inappropriate* ('negative self-concept', 'egocentric' and 'bizarre'). They coded staff responses as *positive attention* (approval, agreement, acceptance, compliments, laughter, prompts for further ordinary interaction); *negative attention* (disapproval, disagreement, rejection, derogatory comments about the speaker); and *ignore* (no response although someone within 6ft of the speaker). They found that staff allocated their attention according to the pattern of percentages shown in Table 5.1.

Table 5.1: Type of Attention Given to Patterns of Behaviour: Percentage of Total Attention

		(rows sum to 100%)
	Positive attention	Negative attention	Ignore
Appropriate behaviour	100	0	0
Neutral behaviour	70.5	1.5	28.0
Inappropriate behaviour	97.3	0	2.7

Source after Sanson-Fisher & Poole, 1980

In other words, staff were almost totally indiscriminate in giving positive attention to behaviour whether appropriate or neutral. It should be noted that the entirely verbal definition of appropriate behaviour, and the highly practical or non-verbal definition of neutral behaviour, account for the zero proportion of *ignore* for appropriate behaviour, while neutral behaviour was ignored 28 per cent of the time. However, the important finding is the lack of discrimination between *appropriate* and *inappropriate* behaviour. In our study (Cullen *et al.*, 1983) in an institution for mentally handicapped people, we used a very similar methodology, except that, following Wolfensberger (1972, 1980) we defined appropriateness/inappropriateness in terms of whether the behaviour is positively or negatively valued in our culture. We found that staff (when they did interact) did not discriminate between appropriate and inappropriate behaviour — they gave positive attention indiscriminately. In terms of social learning theory, then, we would not predict that the residents would themselves have any way of discriminating between appropriate and inappropriate behaviour. Similar phenomena can readily be observed in general hospital wards: in a context characterised by short staffing, and the predominantly medical definitions of needs, it is difficult for patients to acquire more than a modicum of interaction from staff, except by being obstreperous.

Even given this very minimal definition of an appropriate interaction, then, we find no evidence that interactions do have appropriate content. In the Sanson-Fisher and Poole study, in fact, 70 per cent of staff had said they did not believe that inappropriate behaviour should receive positive attention. In our setting there had been much discussion about the role of attention in maintaining undesirable behaviours. Sanson-Fisher and Poole (1980) suggest that this finding of apparently extreme tolerance and encouragement of inappropriate behaviour, is attributable to the medical model of mental illness that pervades such settings. People with mental disorder are seen as 'ill'. They are therefore not responsible for their behaviour and so escape its customary social sanctions. A similar ideology informs the behaviour of some staff in mental handicap services: the handicapped adult is seen as childlike and/or ill, and therefore it is 'not fair', or even 'cruel' to expect them to take any responsibility — they are therefore seen as requiring nursing care, and at the same time denied the exercise of autonomy and choice.

So far, then, we have argued that, even given a very minimal definition of appropriate content of interaction, studies in hospital environments for people with very different disabling conditions do not provide for interactions of appropriate content. It is also possible to devise a less mechanistic and more everyday way of defining appropriate content in interactions. Such a definition also takes in the complete range of settings, whether or not the clients/patients have some sort of mental/behavioural disability/disorder. This is to base the definition of appropriate content on values such as respect, honesty, friendliness and openness. Such a definition would also fit in many ways with at least some approaches to counselling (e.g. humanistic approaches). Hospital environments, hospital culture and many of the features that spill over into the community health services, are largely inimical to these values.

One way of approaching this issue is to ask the question, 'what features of health service culture are likely to influence (positively or negatively) the appropriateness of the content of interactions to the needs of the service user?' For the purposes of this chapter, three such aspects of health service culture will be discussed,

(1) the physical definition of needs,

(2) professional role distance, and

(3) the special physical environment.

Need Definition

The 'medical model' has frequently been criticised as an inadequate approach to problems of mental disorder or mental handicap. However, there are also good reasons for criticising it as an approach to physical illness. At this point we need to state which medical models, or which features of medical models, are up for criticism. The central problem is perhaps the way human beings are seen narrowly as medical entities which sometimes go wrong and need fixing. Those which cannot be fixed through medical technology are of less interest. This ideology is closely bound up with an approach to science and enquiry known variously as scientism, empiricism, positivism or mechanical materialism. It is also closely connected with the dominance of the male-dominated medical profession over other groups of human service workers (e.g. nurses, social workers, physiotherapists) who might otherwise contribute alternative analyses, but who within the present medically defined health service (which includes the processes of training), work largely within that framework.

Seeing people in these physical terms biases the way health and illness are understood, the way in which the various causes of illness are given differing emphases and finally the way in which treatments and prevention are developed. For our purposes, however, the medical model has implications for the way a person who is a patient is likely to be seen.

The medical view sees the sick person as a physical entity, as, for example, 'the chest in bed 5' or 'the appendix who came in last night'. The priorities within the medically-defined health service culture, then, are to attend to the physical aspects of the person, ignoring the economic, social or psychological aspects, or at best hiving some of them off to hospital social workers and dealing with the rest incidentally in a rather random fashion. Indeed, the person's needs are not likely to be seen as primarily to do with how they feel, or what they want, except in so far as these can be seen in medical terms (the response might be a painkiller or valium). (See Figlio (1978); Taussig (1980), for detailed discussion of this aspect of medical ideology.)

For staff working within a system that sees its clients in this way, who have themselves been taught this way of seeing, it can be very difficult to break out of it. The very routines and the system of thinking within the service setting are likely to take more than a little social skills training to change. Incidentally, while the nursing process has been hailed as a way of returning the human individual to the forefront, it is implemented within this highly medically defined culture, and can at best be seen as only part of a strategy for change; this may correspond to the more cynical, but I believe widely held view, that the nursing process makes a fetish of (inappropriate) assessment that leads nowhere — where could it lead in the environment described here?

Professional Roles

As Navarro (1977) has pointed out, the British class system is re-produced within the NHS, with a clear status hierarchy from consultants, through administrators and paramedics, via nurses to ancillary staff. Not only are these groups demarcated from one another, but they also take pains to demarcate themselves very clearly from the users of the service, the patients. There are various ways in which nurses maintain their (chronically threatened — see May and Kelly (1982)) status in relation to patients. Uniforms are an obvious one, with differentiations between ranks to an extent that would be remarkable even in a military context. It has been observed by many people how the abolition of uniforms, for example, in psychiatric hospitals, is often followed by the sprouting of surrogate status badges such as key rings worn on the belt. Similarly, I have caught myself clutching my HMSO diary as an emblem of my status at times when I could not possibly need it, no doubt to maintain my own role differentiation from clients or other staff. Territory is another way of differentiating professional status from patient status. The nursing station is an obvious example, one whose function remains the same even when it is moved out into the ward itself.

All this effort to demarcate staff or professional status from user or patient status is not without its effect on interactions. Put simply, it is difficult to have interactions characterised by respect, honesty, friendliness or openness, when one of the parties (the one with the greater power in the interaction) is striving to establish and to maintain status. This is not just a problem for nurses — my own profession, psychology, is bedevilled by it too — but there is a chronic need of nurses to establish status, because in most health care contexts they are by definition subsidiary to other professional groups in the NHS class system. Again, interpersonal skills training can only alert people to some of the issues in interaction; it does not change the context within which interaction occurs. Indeed, some themes in traditional social skills training based on Argyle (1969) (e.g. its goal-orientated nature) are

actually consistent with the type of professional role distance discussed here.

Special Environments

Hospitals are strange places where strange things happen to people. A
ward, whether surgical, medical, psychiatric or whatever, has no clear
counterpart or analogue in the ordinary world. Some aspects of its
alienating nature such as the lack of defensible space, have been
documented in the literature of environmental psychology (see Kagan
and Burton (1982) for a brief review). However, the strangeness of the
hospital setting is so immense that it almost defies analysis, yet because
hospitals do exist, and they are places that are in many ways highly
respected by the public, we often fail to label them in this way. Instead
we seem to take the ward environment for granted — as part of the real
world — rather than as an incredible aberration when viewed from the
standpoint of our everyday life in houses, offices, factories, pubs and
the like.

The hospital, then, presents a triumph of 'deculturation'. By going
into it, we go from the familiar places where our interpersonal skills
work, into an unfamiliar environment where they have lost many of
their natural setting events. One way of seeing this is to ask the question:
'What is the appropriate way to have an ordinary conversation in a
hospital ward?' In ordinary environments, the features of the environment often define appropriateness: conversation is integrated into a fab-
ric of interaction with each other, and with the physical environment. In
an ordinary workplace we have to talk about aspects of the job, and we
may use supports such as the newspaper or a radio playing to start off
conversations about current affairs, or sport, the Royal Family or other
trivia. At home, the tasks involved in running the home and catering for
the children, the cat, or the garden will similarly set off conversation and
other social interaction that is appropriate to (or at least modulated by)
the changing pattern of needs of the participants.

The hospital is different. As anyone who has visited someone in
hospital knows, it is often really difficult to converse appropriately. In
these decultured environments there is nothing to talk about, apart from
topics like the reason for being there (a bit sensitive to fill up much of the
time), the other people there (a bit taboo, especially since they might
overhear), the meals (safe but boring) or events outside the ward (again
a bit sensitive since the patient is excluded from them). Interaction

assumes an uneasy, staccato manner for both patient and visitor, however well they know each other. The argument then is that these problems also beset the people who work in these strange places, especially since interaction is a two-way process. In a radically unnatural context, skilled interaction is likely to break down because the usual props provided in ordinary places, are missing.

Conclusions

The contention, then, is that the environments of the health service are structured, both physically and socially, in ways that militate against there being 'good interactions' from the points of view of the users of the service. Commonly, the opportunities for interaction are too few, they tend to be too brief, and several forces, both structural and ideological, work against their having an appropriate content.

If the situation is to be improved, it will not be as a result of first blaming nurses for lack of skill and then training them in it. It will instead require a major restructuring of the environments and culture of health care, a restructuring that must tackle professionalism, medical definitions of health, and as far as is possible the dominance of the hospital in health care provision.

References

Argyle, (1969) *Social Interaction*, Methuen: London

Ayllon, T. and Michael, J. (1959) 'The Psychiatric Nurse as a Behavioral Engineer', *Journal of the Experimental Analysis of Behavior*, 2, 323-34

Blackman, D.K., Howe, M. and Pinkston, E.M. (1976) 'Increasing Participation in the Social Interaction of the Institutionalized Elderly', *The Gerontologist*, 16, 69-76

Burton, M. (1979) 'The Use of Feedback of Observational Data to Promote Change in Occupational Therapy in a Psychogeriatric Ward', unpublished MSc thesis, University of Manchester

Burton, M. (1980) 'Evaluation and Change in a Psychogeriatric Ward through Direct Observation and Feedback', *British Journal of Psychiatry*, 137, 566-71

Cullen, C., Burton M., Watts, S. and Thomas, M. (1983) 'A Preliminary Report on the Nature of Interactions in a Mental Handicap Institution', *Behaviour Research and Therapy*, 21, 579-83

Figlio, K. (1978) 'Chlorosis and Chronic Disease in 19th-century Britain: the social constitution of somatic illness in a capitalist society', *International Journal of Health Services*, 8, 589-617

Fox, W. (1983) 'Staff and Patient Behaviour Profiles on Long Stay/Rehabilitation Psychiatric Wards'. Paper presented to British Psychological Society: London

Gelfand, D.M., Gelfand, S. and Dobson, W.R. (1967) 'Unprogrammed Reinforcement of Patients' Behaviour in a Mental Hospital', *Behaviour Research and Therapy*, 201-7

Grant, G.W.B. (1974) 'An examination of Care Patterns in Subnormality Hospitals with differing Resource Levels', unpublished doctoral thesis, University of Manchester Institute of Science and Technology

Holahan, C.J. (1979) 'Redesigning Physical Environments to Enhance Social Interactions' in R.F. Muñoz, L.R. Snowden, J.G. Kelly and Associates, *Social and Psychological Research in Community Settings*, Jossey-Bass: San Francisco

Kagan, C. and Burton, M. (1982) 'Scenes of Improvement', *Nursing Mirror*, *155*, 44-5

Macleod Clark, J. (1984) 'Verbal Communication in Nursing' in A. Faulkner (ed.), *Recent Advances in Nursing*, *7*, *Communication*, Churchill Livingstone: Edinburgh

May, D. and Kelly, M.P. (1982) 'Chancers, Pests and Poor Wee Souls : problems of legitimation in psychiatric nursing', *Sociology of Health and Illness*, *4*, 279-301

Navarro, V. (1977) *Class Struggle, the State and Medicine: an Historical and Contemporary Analysis of the Medical Sector in Great Britain*, Martin Robertson: London

Porterfield, J., Blunden, R. and Blewitt, E. (1980) 'Improving Environments for Profoundly Handicapped Adults — Using Prompts and Social Attention to Maintain High Group Engagement, *Behavior Modification*, *4*, 225-41

Sanson-Fisher, R.W. and Poole, A.D. (1980) 'The Content of Interactions : naturally occurring contingencies within a short-stay psychiatric unit', *Advances in Behaviour Research and Therapy*, *2*, 145-57

Sanson-Fisher, R.W., Poole, A.D. and Thompson, V. (1979) 'Behaviour Patterns Within a General Hospital Psychiatric Unit : an observational study', *Behaviour Research and Therapy*, *17*, 317-32

Taussig, M. (1980) 'Reification and the Consciousness of the Patient', *Social Science and Medicine*, *14B*, 3-13

Wolfensberger, W. (with others) (1972) *The Principle of Normalization in Human Services*, National Institute on Mental Retardation: Toronto

Wolfensberger, W. (1980) 'A Brief Overview of the Principle of Normalization' in R.J. Flynn & K.E. Nitsch (eds), *Normalization, Social Integration and Community Services*, University Park Press: Baltimore, Maryland

Zimring, C., Weitzer, W. and Knight, R.C. (1982) 'Opportunity for Control and the Designed Environment: the case of an institution for the developmentally disabled' in A. Baum and J.E. Singer (eds) *Advances in Environmental Psychology, Vol. 4*, Erlbaum: Hillside, New Jersey

6 THE WIDER SOCIAL CONTEXT OF INTERPERSONAL SKILLS IN NURSING

Francis Lillie

Introduction

In the previous two chapters Mark Burton and Ann Faulkner have suggested that environmental and organisational contexts must be considered when interpersonal skills in nursing are examined and when any attempt to change (improve) those skills is made. The environment and the organisation both impose constraints on the effective use of interpersonal skill and on any change programme. However, both the immediate environment and the organisation of nursing practice are part of a much wider social, political and economic context, at any point in history. In order to appreciate fully the use and misuse of interpersonal skill as displayed by individual people, it is necessary to consider this wider social context, which, inevitably, will be linked to specific cultures (or, in this sense, nation states with governmental policies relating to the funding and organisation of health services).

This chapter attempts to fit interpersonal skills and nursing into the context of the health care system of the United Kingdom. Before this is attempted it is worth noting briefly the pessimistic *world* context of our time.

The World Context

In the widest world context many members of the caring professions are dominated by the probable extinction of the human race by nuclear weapons. *The Fate of the Earth*, as Schell (1982) dramatically called his summary of the evidence for the probable annihilation of human, animal and plant life, is bleak. It seems unlikely that the largest caring profession in the world will have much to do after a nuclear holocaust for, as American ex-president Jimmy Carter has said, 'The survivors, if any, would live in despair amid the poisoned ruins of a civilisation that had committed suicide.' More immediately, today, famine and disease ravage many nations where there is little medical or nursing support. These facts may have a direct influence on nurses' (and patients') morale, which will affect the quality of their interpersonal relations. In addition, vital energy and resources may be taken up opposing promoting the use of nuclear weapons and/or challenging/advocating a nursing response to the effects of nuclear warfare.

Narrowing the focus, I would remind the reader of the large range of health care systems and different economic and political contexts around the world. While they are complex and varied, and while comparisons are difficult, these different systems should prompt the reader to examine his/her own political and economic value system in relation to nursing. For instance, within the Soviet Union there is very good evidence of the abuse of patients' rights and imprisonment of patients by doctors, nurses and other professionals. In the UK abuse is not directed by central government, but the sins of omission and commission of long stay institutions are catalogued in government enquiries into appalling conditions of neglect. This has led to an increased awareness of patients' rights and concern at neglect in the three priority client care groups in the NHS — mentally ill people, mentally handicapped people and elderly people. A political and economic analysis is relevant also to general nursing, outside those priority areas (see Doyal, 1979). For instance, an analysis of current USA nursing practices shows that sometimes diagnostic procedures and treatments are performed for the practitioner's profit at the expense of the patient's health needs. Within Africa, mothers have been persuaded not to breast-feed their children and to give them powdered milk. This practice has been detrimental to their babies' health, but has led to healthy profits for the particular multinational company. Many international examples such as these are available from Health Action International or the International Organisation of Consumers' Unions (The Health Services, 1983). Generally in the Western world (including the UK) tobacco and alcohol consumption is encouraged by companies which harm individuals and the health of the society at large. The development of health (and illness) systems is frequently seen to be due to political pressures external to the health needs of the population (e.g. Doyal, 1979). This, too, makes individual responses to patients' needs by nurses difficult to achieve: often, with the best will in the world, nurses are unable to implement the interpersonal changes they see to be necessary, due to these external (political) pressures.

Health Care Funding

I am well aware that there is a range of different methods of funding health care that makes international comparisons difficult, since I have worked and lived with different health care systems in New Zealand, America and the UK but my intention at the beginning of this chapter is that each reader should examine his or her own reaction to the wider context of the health system in order to reach some ethical equanimity, with a useful question always hanging on the lips, 'What if it were me, or mine?' For instance, I can summarise my own concern by asking this question of you, the reader, as if I were speaking to you. How would you feel if your child, bleeding from the face, was turned away from a sumptuously equipped health facility in one of the richest cities in the world because you had too little cash in your pocket? This actual example from Los Angeles clarifies for many people the whole point of free service at the moment of 'acute' human need which the NHS actually delivers. This brief mention of the nature of health care funding is relevant to the UK context in the 1980s with an increase in privatisation of services. It is worth reminding the reader that the Royal Commission on the National Health Service advised against privatisation:

> We are not convinced that the claimed advantages of insurance, finance or substantial increases in charge revenue would outweigh their undoubted disadvantages in terms of equity and administrative costs. The same disadvantages arise from the existing NHS charges. (Report of the Royal Commission, 1979, p.353)

Partial privatisation, or contracting out, has, indeed, been costly as Paul (1984) documents with reference to one example of this practice.

Policy regarding funding may have other direct and indirect consequences for the interpersonal nursing context. Reductions in funding may mean staff shortages which in turn may lead to greater stress and likelihood that staff will experience 'burnout' with its concomitant implications for interpersonal relations with patients and colleagues (McIntee and Firth, 1984). Furthermore, patients in overcrowded outpatients' clinics or experiencing long delays in receiving treatment may become impatient or aggressive; their behaviour will demand particular interpersonal skills of nurses — possibly placatory rather than facilitative skills! Similarly, nurses may feel constrained in their replies to patients' questions such as 'Is there nothing that can be done?', when they know the test/procedure has been 'cut' with reductions in the budget. Morale may be seriously affected by funding cuts as unemployment reaches qualified staff, or yet another reorganisation of the NHS means that job choice for many nurses is restricted. Low morale and uncertainty lead to poor job satisfaction and have a detrimental influence on the effective use of interpersonal skills (see Chapter 3, by Peter Banister and Carolyn Kagan).

The NHS System

Thus far the reader has been reminded of the harsh reality of the wider context for nurses. There is no environmental vacuum for an illness or a patient (as we shall call in this chapter the person in need of help, care or attention). These first paragraphs also lead to the basic thesis of this chapter: *that we professionals have to acknowledge this wider context and integrate our consumer/personal selves with our producer/ professional selves.* We have to compare what we (ourselves, our families, friends and neighbours) *want* when we seek information and advice on health, with what we *receive* from the service that pays our salaries and over which we have some degree of control. Hopefully the perspective on your own health care, which would include your social context, your living arrangement or family circumstances, would be very similar to the perspective that you would use to view any patient in your care. This wider social perspective is emphasised, as often in general hospital nursing nurses have been taught and dominated by medical and nursing professions which have exaggerated the scientific basis of high technology medicine. This teaching has frequently ignored information on the social and psychological variables involved in 'human' presentation of physical illness, mental illness or distress. In addition, the predominant approach to interpersonal skills in nursing is a psychological one, which stresses the importance of the *individual* (nurse, patient, relative etc.) for effective interpersonal skill. This chapter is about not ignoring the wider social context of the patient, the staff and the structure of the NHS.

There are four problematic aspects of the NHS system, analyses of which will serve to give the reader a critical perspective of the wider context of interpersonal skills. These are:
(1) the medical domination of the health system; (2) the language that communicates images to the health workers and their patients; (3) the secrecy that characterises national and local NHS policy making, and

the consequent lack of consultation of the consumer in decision-making processes; and (4) the problem of access to health advice and care for the priority groups. I intend to review these aspects, and then to argue that there is a need to strengthen the education of the community (including nurses and doctors) so that people can obtain most health advice and care comprehensively at a local level.

Medical Domination of the Health System

The first aspect to review is that of medical power, and for a full analysis the reader is referred to Ham (1982) where the domination of professionals (largely doctors) rather than consumers over control of health care is well documented. As Ham (1982, p.86) says:

> Consumer groups are heavily dependent on the advice, information and expertise they have to offer, and cannot threaten sanctions in the same way as producer groups.

Similarly, Brown, another writer on health policy, says:

> the machinery on the health and welfare side of DHSS tends to be dominated by those who provide service rather than those for whom the services are intended (Ham, 1982, p.193)

Ham summarises well the historical roots of this domination by

> physicians, surgeons, and apothecaries in winning state approval for their position, and in turning their occupations into professions having exclusive control over their area of work. Medical dominance does not imply a conspiracy against subordinate groups. Rather, it reflects the power of doctors, their control of key resources such as expertise and knowledge, and their ability to achieve acceptance for their own concept of health. (Ham, 1982, p.161)

Ham's analysis here is a moderate viewpoint of the contemporary scene, avoiding a simple conspiracy way of viewing medical hegemony. This medical (and sometimes associated nursing) domination makes change, from an interpersonal skills perspective, difficult because the medical profession is established and the *status quo* protects their interests. For some concrete examples of how this medical dominance can directly affect the effective use of interpersonal skills by nurses, see the discussions of Peter Banister and Carolyn Kagan (Chapter 3) and Ann Faulkner (Chapter 4).

Language and Images

The second aspect to analyse is the language that health professionals use between themselves, with their patients and with the public at large. Sometimes concepts are grossly oversimplified and words are used in false opposition on major policy issues. One such example of this is the use of the terms 'health' and 'illness'. 'Health' suggests a static endpoint to which people can, through the appropriate lifestyle, increase their life-span. 'Illness' has been widely used as a label when there is no organic or physiological dysfunction. This labelling has led to confusion where inappropriate characteristics associated with people are labelled as illness because they are apparently unusual or undesirable in that social context. For instance homosexuality was once seen as an illness by professions, when clearly it reflects nothing more than a particular sexual preference. Pregnancy, too, is still frequently treated as an 'illness' when it generally represents a normal and healthy course of events (Roberts, 1982).

Sometimes NHS language seems deliberately impersonal, perhaps to distance staff from the impact of administrative expediency. For example, in NHS planning, beds 'silt up' if people stay too long in their hospital beds, or, patients are 'decanted' from one ward to another if they are moved from one ward to another as a group. While health planners do not think of the patients as mud or vintage port, there is a danger for us all that the language will allow us to gloss over the individual medical and social circumstances of people silting up beds or being decanted from one ward to another. Impersonality is reinforced by clinicians who 'label'. Sometimes people are solely identified by a portion of their anatomy, condition, illness or age. So 'she's a geri'., 'the ulcerated leg in bed 4', and 'the schizophrenic in bed 5' are all professionally *unacceptable* shorthand descriptions which allow clinicians to distance themselves from the person's distress and dilemma. Furthermore, these shorthand terms lead to a failure in logical and scientific thinking. The professional labelling of such groups as 'epileptics' or 'schizophrenics' is relatively meaningless and diminishes understanding. The term 'epileptics' does not refer to a group of people with anything very significant in common. Two people suffering from epilepsy may or may not be taking anti-convulsants, and they may or may not have abnormal EEGs. 'Schizophrenics' as a label is also relatively useless. One-third of people who experience an episode of schizophrenia recover completely and they are indistinguishable from you or from me. More damagingly, it must be pointed out that shorthand terms like 'geri'. or 'schizo' become denigrating terms and eventually are epithets of abuse.

Sometimes particular language powerfully reinforces stereotypes in official documents. One of the largest Regions in the NHS is currently proudly reporting on 'Accommodation for mentally ill people', which implies that people who are mentally ill (which is the minimally correct way of putting the expression) are always to be identified by the hybrid phrase with its elements pessimistically inseparable. Actually, even people with the most serious 'mental illness' such as schizophrenia have *episodes* of the acute symptoms (that lead to the diagnosis).

The fact that our use of language creates and reinforces negative attitudes, which in turn affect our use of interpersonal skill, is demonstrated by the normalisation literature (for example, O'Brien and Tyne, 1981). The ideology of normalisation emphasises the need to use ordinary means of care delivery to reduce the isolation and segregation from the ordinary community of people who are impaired or disadvantaged. The most graphic normalisation example for me is the continued use of mini-buses labelled, for example, 'Mentally Handicapped, Gift of Swaggertown Businessman's Guild'. Would the reader like to be driven around his/her community by a driver in a bus labelled 'Nurse with Piles'? This example, along with the continued use of terms like 'subnormal' or 'mongol' (neither of which should be used), makes the point of how language, image and attitudes can bias our perspective of thousands of people for whom we are supposed to care.

Secrecy of Policy Making

The third aspect of the wider context to review is that of the secrecy that characterises much of the decision making about health policy. A recent editorial, 'Evasive Tactics', in a leading journal *(Health and Social Services Journal,* 1984), reminds us that key DHSS circulars and documents are not available as and when they should be. Secrecy about health issues nationally and locally is currently being challenged by consumer organisations (see, for example, Intercom, 1984) who believe that people should generally have access to policy documents that concern their health. The Community Health Councils were set up in 1974 as statutory watchdogs but they have few teeth and have had to battle over the subsequent decade to be consulted by Health Authorities: furthermore, it has been argued that their composition does not reflect the communities they represent (Doyal, 1979). (There have been similar difficulties for consumers in gaining access to planning and service information from Social Services, although of course the latter's local accountability to local political processes sometimes is used to challenge their right to secrecy.) Since development of community care is likely to depend strongly on cooperation between the two arms of the DHSS body, this communication gap needs to be closed. Unfortunately mutual trust between doctors and other professionals is not helped by the infamous and secret merit (distinction) awards to some medical Consultants. These awards, which can mean as much as £22,390 on a basic salary of £20,200 for some Consultants, are suspected of being granted to those who do not threaten or challenge current clinical practice. I do not argue with the particular sums, only with the fact that the merit list of names is secret, whereas a senior nurse's salary, or the author's, is a matter of public knowledge. This kind of secrecy hardly helps modern multidisciplinary team work with its emphasis on sharing and trust, an emphasis that is particularly marked (though not exclusively so) with reference to the priority client groups.

Secrecy is also a characteristic of the pharmaceutical industry, where naturally the commercial nature of the operations demands it to some degree. Clearly there is conflict here between a patient's or a society's right to know, and, the rights of commercial organisations. A commentator (Openmind, 1984) has recently criticised the way the cost to the NHS of medication is protected by the Official Secrets Act, when the pharmaceutical industry itself is fully aware of its own profit margins. There seems little reason to withhold this information from the public. Of course, the largest category of NHS prescription drugs is that of psychotropic drugs, and in this area there are non-drug alternatives, with good scientific evidence of effectiveness from various psychological therapies. The commercial pressures exerted by the pharmaceutical industry in making these drugs available and in persuading practitioners to use them may, by default, prohibit the development of therapeutic interpersonal skills.

While some of this secrecy is deliberate, to maintain the commercial and professional *status quo*, there is a considerable failure to inform that arises from motives of goodwill and protective (often interfering) concern. Traditional medical and nursing people have thought that experts know best and that treatment compliance is more likely if the patient is not involved. This naive professional autonomy has prevented patients from knowing the full facts (as they are known) about their own bodies and minds. Sometimes the individual patient, patient group or society at large colludes in this policy and prefers not to know details about their illness or state of health. While clinical examples can occasionally be quoted to support an approach with concealment of the truth from distressed patients who are very ill or dying, these are *exceptions* to the general need for the public to know, and for the public to have access to medical and nursing information.

Access to Health Information, Advice and Care

The recognition of the need for information to be public has increased through various pressure groups and the media, with attacks on professional labelling, the lack of information available to the individual in the clinical situation and the lack of consumer involvement in planning. For instance, a District's Health Care Planning Team for the Elderly frequently may have no representative of large and influential voluntary organisations such as Age Concern, or a District's Mental Illness Planning Team may have no community representative. When professional people on these committees *are* elderly or, for instance, *have* experienced mental illness themselves, they are seldom able to use this information and integrate their professional and personal roles. The widespread stigma of mental illness and the tendency for professionals not to self-disclose their personal selves makes it difficult for a District Treasurer or a District Psychologist to say at a meeting: 'With my depression I gained considerably from occupational therapy and therefore I think we need to look at the funding of that department.' On the other hand it is easier for either senior officer to comment publicly on when he broke a leg and how effective occupational therapy was at that time. Until professionals at all levels feel (and are) free to disclose their personal stake in health care, they will be party to propagating the conventional wisdom that patients are sick and thereby deviant and thus have little to say regarding the reality of their condition, other than to describe symptoms. Nurses, doctors and other 'health professionals', are not sick, not deviant and are thereby in a position to assess the health needs of their (deviant) patients. This mutual pretence puts intolerable burdens on those nurses and patients who attempt to relate to each other in interpersonally honest ways.

I have suggested above that there is a continuum of access to health information (at policy and clinical levels) ranging from deliberate secrecy controlled by vested interests to lack of consultation with the client care groups which is often caused by professional ignorance. It is not surprising, then, that reduction in disadvantage and stigma and increase in resources for the three NHS priority groups have been slow. While the elderly and those people categorised as mentally ill and mentally handicapped have been recognised as priority groups for a decade, it is important to emphasise that other people are subject to widespread inequalities in *access* to health-giving environments, health education and health care. This evidence is summarised by Townsend and Davidson (1982), who present the findings of the 'Black Report'. People of other categories, such as racial minorities and the poor, are discriminated against to varying extents depending on particular local health delivery systems and particular socioeconomic environments. These comments on race and poverty will be briefly qualified.

Firstly, on racial discrimination the reader is referred to McNaught (1984). Recently there has been widespread concern in ethnic minority groups when, in 1982, the Government decided to charge overseas visitors using the NHS, as this entailed checking 'visible' minorities and residents with foreign-sounding names. Since then the revenue obtained from overseas visitors has been less than the increased cost of administering the system. Indeed, Gordon (1983) goes so far as to suggest that medical techniques and examinations have played an important part in immigration control in Britain, in those situations where no question of health is involved. Secondly, there is a burgeoning literature concerning the links between poverty, ill health and access to care exemplified in the writings of Professor Peter Townsend (for instance, Townsend, 1983). There is little doubt that a major review is necessary if the impact of benefits in the incredibly complex welfare system of Health and Social Service policy is to lead to an equitable system for those who are temporarily or chronically ill. To understand the tragic problems within the benefit system of people who are disabled demands that the reader have direct current clinical experience of these problems or read published verbatim reports, (for instance, Blaxter, 1976).

Furthermore community care usually means women rather than men as constant carers for disabled people and chronically ill people in the community (Finch and Groves, 1983). Women are usually unacknowledged and unpaid in this role, and this needs recognition in any review of the benefits system.

Implications for an Interpersonal Skills Approach to Health Care

Given these wider aspects of the NHS system, what is the way forwards if nursing is to use an interpersonal skills approach to health care? There will need to be wholehearted liaison between Health and Social Services at planning and service levels. Health care in the next decade for defined priority groups and other people will depend particularly on the staff of community or primary care services being appropriately educated. All community staff will have to cope with the psychological and social characteristics of general medical practice that have become increasingly recognised. The NHS should develop comprehensive health education and facilitate self-help groups which will enable people to take more control over some of their own health needs. This may involve the public lowering their expectations of easy or lasting cure by medication. So, in addition to professionals needing a radical re-training programme, the public will have to change their expectations or attitudes to health care. To some extent this process is under way in the women's health movement (Doyal, 1983). Because of the four aspects reviewed above, considerable leadership will have to come from the health professionals if an interpersonal skills approach to health care is to succeed. The community re-education process is further hindered by the lack of time for health debates in this society at the level of Parliament (see, for instance, Solesbury, 1976).

Furthermore there is likely to be powerful opposition from the pharmaceutical industry which is generally opposed to the education of professionals in the social and psychological causes and manifestations of illness. Drug companies' involvement in medical education has recently been criticised by Professor Rawlins, a Professor of Clinical Pharmacology at the University of Newcastle:

Doctors are becoming so accustomed to sponsored postgraduate education that it is difficult to attract them to meetings where they have to pay for their own registration and refreshments. (Rawlins, 1984, p.277)

In addition, doctors are not immune from propaganda. Professor Rawlins reminds us:

The harsh truth is that not one of us is impervious to the promotional activities of the industry, and the industry uses its various techniques because they are very effective. (Rawlins, 1984, p.277)

There is one drug representative for every seven GPs and they operate like any other group of sophisticated sales people who have comprehensive personal files on their targets (doctors) so as to help persuade them of the worth of their company's products. This is one of the factors that has no doubt led to over-prescription, for instance, of tranquillisers (Melville, 1984; Tyrer, Owen and Dawling, 1983). One of the national problems is that GPs have had no financial limit on their prescribing practices unlike medical consultants in the hospital service who have had relatively controlled budgets. As this book goes to press, the Government is investigating this open-ended aspect of Family Practitioner budgets.

Nevertheless, to be positive, in an interpersonal skills manner, there are some ways forwards. Staff will have to integrate their personal selves and what health advice and care they want, with their professional selves, as deliverers of the service. Staff will have to seek out information and good health practices; such a re-education will involve them in knowing of good local and national practices. For instance in mental health there is an organisation called Good Practices in Mental Health that publishes a guide for organising local studies (GPMH, 1980). Furthermore journals such as the *Health and Social Services Journal*, and *Critical Social Policy* report on innovative schemes which, whilst not necessarily 'scientifically' validated, suggest novel ways of approaching different health problems and client groups. The problem of validation is for the evaluators, not the innovators.

Education will also involve nurses in abandoning their traditional distance from their patients and adopting an enabling function, with an interpersonal skills approach, to the patients. For instance health visitors should be able to facilitate community support (De'Ath, 1982), and should perhaps run 'drop in' centres on an informal basis for children instead of the traditional child health clinics (Field *et al.*, 1982). This would have enormous implications for changes in the nature of, and possibilities for, effective use of interpersonal skills. Finally, at the same time as people put forward positive suggestions and applaud good practices, they will have to challenge the negative aspects that have been reviewed above *wherever* they meet them, whether at an individual professional, ward or committee level.

Summary

This chapter has considered four critical aspects of the wider social context of nursing and health care delivery. Brief reviews were made of the medical domination of the health system; the language used to communicate images by and to health workers and their patients; the secrecy that characterises national and local NHS policy making and consequent lack of consultation of the consumer; and the problem of access to health advice and care for the priority and other disadvantaged groups. It was argued that this wider context can have both indirect and direct effects on the effective use of interpersonal skill. The socio/political context can affect nurses' (and other health workers', and patients') morale, and thus, indirectly their effective use of interpersonal skill: furthermore, role distance created between professionals because of the way the NHS is structured (and re-organised) may adversely affect interpersonal relations between health workers. In addition, the creation of health and illness images, through the language we use, dictates attitudes to and of nurses, which, too, may constrain their freedom to engage clinically and personally valuable interpersonal skill.

Policy decisions, influenced by, for example, Central Government, the medical establishment or the pharmaceutical industry, may have direct consequences for the deployment of effective and therapeutically beneficial interpersonal skill. The control wielded by these bodies may make individual (or local) attempts to change interpersonal nursing practices extremely difficult.

It was suggested, though, that there is room for optimism. If health care professionals recognise that they are also consumers of the health service, and attempt to integrate their personal selves with their professional selves, they will begin to challenge the socio/political/ economic *status quo* of their work. Too often, nurses do not critically examine the wider context of their nursing practices and thus they (and others) do not realise the challenge before them. The challenge has to be accepted as a patient, as a staff member and above all else as a citizen concerned with the basic human right of health care. In the final analysis, there is a moral imperative on us to use all three roles in furthering a humane, interpersonal skills approach to health care services.

Acknowledgements

These are due to Mrs Sarah Sexton for the efficient typing of various drafts.

References

Blaxter, M. (1976) *The Meaning of Disability*, Heinemann: London

De'Ath, E. (1982) 'A Preventive Approach to Family Life: The role of the Health Visitor', *Health Visitor*, 55, 282-4

Doyal, L. (1979) *The Political Economy of Health*, Pluto: London (with I. Pennell)

Doyal, L. (1983) 'Women, Health and the Sexual Division of Labour: A case study of the women's health movement in Britain', *Critical Social Policy*, *3*, 21-34

Field, S., Draper, J., Kerr, M., and Hare, M. (1982) 'A Consumer View of the Health Visiting Service', *Health Visitor*, 55, 229-301

Finch, J. and Groves, D. (eds) (1983) *A Labour of Love: Women, Work and Caring*, Routledge and Kegan Paul: London

GPMH (1980) *Good Practices in Mental Health: A guide for organising local studies*, International Hospital Federation: London

Gordon, P. (1983) 'Medicine, Racism and Immigration Control', *Critical Social Policy*, *3*, 6-20

Ham, C. (1982) *Health Policy in Britain*, Macmillan: London

Health and Social Services Journal (1984), *XCIV, 4910*, p.961. Editorial: 'Evasive Tactics'

The Health Services (1983) *No. 45*, 25 March, p.12

Intercom (1984) No. 52, March, MIND: London

McIntee, J. and Firth, H. (1984) 'How to Beat the Burnout', *Health and Social Services Journal,* 9 February, 166-8

McNaught, A. (1984) *Race and Health Care in the UK*, CHEMS, Polytechnic of the South Bank: London

Melville, J. (1984) *The Tranquilliser Trap*, Fontana: London

O'Brien, J. and Tyne, A. (1981) *The Principle of Normalisation: A Foundation for Effective Services*, Community and Mental Handicap Educational and Research Association: London

Openmind (1984) *No. 9*, June/July, p.13, MIND: London

Paul, J. (1984) 'Contracting Out in the NHS : Can we afford to take the risk?' *Critical Social Policy*, *4*, 83-92

Rawlins, M.D. (1984) 'Doctors and the Drug Makers', *The Lancet*, 4 August, p.276

Report of the Royal Commission on the National Health Service (1979) HMSO : London

Roberts, H. (1982) *Women, Health and Reproduction*, Routledge and Kegan Paul : London

Schell, J. (1982) *The Fate of the Earth*, Picador: London

Solesbury, W. (1976) 'The Environment Agenda', *Public Administration*, Winter, 379-97

Townsend, P. (1983) 'A Theory of Poverty and the Role of Social Policy' In M. Loney, D. Boswell and J. Clarke (eds), *Social Policy and Social Welfare*, Open University Press: Milton Keynes

Townsend, P. and Davidson, N. (1982) *Inequalities in Health (the 'Black Report')*, Penguin: Harmondsworth

Tyrer, P., Owen, R. and Dawling, S. (1983) 'Gradual Withdrawal of Diazepam after Long-term Therapy', *The Lancet*, 25 June, 402-6

PART III:

INTERPERSONAL SKILLS IN PRACTICAL NURSING

EDITORIAL INTRODUCTION

The organisational, environmental and wider social contexts are just some of the factors that influence the effective deployment of interpersonal skills by nurses. However, *Desmond Cormack*, in *Chapter 7*, warns against accepting the 'fact' that nurses do not use effective interpersonal skills. He contends that recognition must be given to the different types of interpersonal skills usage. The use of interpersonal skills is both myth and reality, depending on the type of skill under consideration. Cormack distinguishes between formal/structured interpersonal skills, and less formal, indirect interpersonal skills. He argues that relatively little nurse-patient interaction time is spent in using formal, goal-directed skills, and yet this is the yardstick by which nurses' interpersonal competence is generally evaluated. As nurses' roles develop, they may be required to develop formal, goal-directed interpersonal skills, and this may have implications for training. As it is, though, nurses frequently use less formal indirect interpersonal skills to good effect. They should not, therefore, be continually underselling themselves in terms of their levels of interpersonal skill.

Peter Maguire, however, in *Chapter 8*, points to deficiencies in key interpersonal skills that do, perhaps, blur these distinctions between different types of skill. The assessment of patients' needs frequently requires nurses to detect psychosocial problems if they are to plan for good nursing care. Yet, he argues, nurses are rarely seen to employ those interpersonal skills that will enable them to do this. Maguire also notes that nurses are generally poor at giving information, explanation and reassurance, thus detracting from the quality of nursing care they are able to deliver. He supports his case with examples from recordings of nurse-patient interactions, and just as Desmond Cormack anticipated the need for training in formal, goal-directed interpersonal skills, so Peter Maguire sees training as the solution to interpersonal skill deficiencies.

The particular skill of giving information is the focus of *Bryn Davis'* review in *Chapter 9*. The growing literature on the clinical effect of nurses giving pre-operative information in various forms is examined, with an emphasis on the importance of defining criterion measures of nursing care outcomes. Davis concludes that, in this context, those measures that relate to psychological and physical factors of stress reduction, and that involve information-giving that considers the patients' points of view, are the most valuable. He goes on to describe an implementation project in which nurses participated in planning the study, and that involved ward, administrative and education staff. In this study, nurses collected data as part of their everyday work. The success of the project is seen to illustrate the fact that ordinary nurses can achieve the same results as researchers, a finding which should endorse the call for nursing research to be of greater relevance to practical nurses. Davis stresses the importance of the cooperation between researchers, managers, educators and practitioners for the success of the project, and presents this study as a model of 'good practice'.

7 THE MYTH AND REALITY OF INTERPERSONAL SKILLS USE IN NURSING

Desmond Cormack

Introduction

The use of interpersonal skills in nursing is the concern of *all* nurses working in *all* specialities. Indeed, the work of this profession could not be accomplished without these skills. However, because my major research and clinical background in interpersonal skills use has been in psychiatric nursing, I will draw on that experience in this discussion. More specifically, I will draw on the clinically based research in which I sought to describe the nature and function of psychiatric nursing (see Cormack, 1983). That work, coupled with a long-standing involvement in nursing generally, has resulted in many of the views expressed in this paper. Some of these views are research based, others are anecdotal and experiential.

Psychiatric Nursing Described (Cormack, 1983) is a published version of my doctor of philosophy thesis in which I asked the following questions: First, what do psychiatric nurses do in terms of delivery of effective and ineffective nursing care? This was answered by collecting and analysing 4,477 critical incidents provided by respondents who were mostly nurses but who included a number of doctors and patients. Second, what are psychiatric nurses trained to do? Third, how is their work formally described in terms of a job description? Fourth, which criteria are used to assess the work of the psychiatric nurse?

A major section of that work, 1,497 critical incidents, related to the extent to which the psychiatric nurse 'uses self as a therapeutic tool'. The incidents, which contained significantly more effective than ineffective ones, were equally distributed among *all six* grades of ward-based nursing staff. Two examples illustrate the use of interpersonal skills, one in an effective manner, the other ineffectively.

Effective example. Patient in acute admission ward reporting on a charge nurse:

> One day I felt really confused and depressed, I felt like killing myself.

107

I told one of the nurses how I felt and she sat down with me and had a chat with me. It helped me greatly just being able to talk to someone about how I felt. The nurse had really helped me by just letting me talk. (p.72)

Ineffective example. Patient in acute admission ward reporting on a staff nurse:

There was a time when I was depressed and inwardly crying out for someone to talk to. The staff nurse was not prepared to give up even one minute of her time to discuss my feelings. I know they all do a marvellous job but there are times when you need to talk. (p.72)

These examples are firm evidence of the importance of interpersonal skills use in psychiatric nursing. The fact that both were provided by patients (consumers of nursing care) adds weight to the argument that nurses have an important, positive or negative, contribution to make in this area. Virtually all examples of the effective use of interpersonal skills were of the direct goal (informal) and indirect goal types (see below).

Three further types of data (documentary data) in the form of *job descriptions*, *training schedules* and *assessment criteria* for each grade were collected and analysed. In relation to the use of interpersonal skills, bearing in mind that all grades of ward-based psychiatric nurses were reported as having virtually equally important roles to play, documentary data for all grades were closely examined for reference to interpersonal skills. The general conclusion from the examination was that the subject 'interpersonal skills use', or 'uses self as a therapeutic tool', was prominent by its general absence from either job descriptions, training schedules or assessment criteria. It is encouraging to note that the new RMN training syllabus for England and Wales (General Nursing Council, 1982) includes a range of interpersonal skills, and the 'intentional and conscious use of self' in the Nursing Skills curricula guidelines. Both are seen to be vital for all therapeutic interaction.

Interpersonal Skills

For the purpose of this chapter, 'interpersonal' skills are regarded as being those skills which are used by a person or persons to reach a goal in collaboration with another person or persons. Thus, if I give a pre-operative patient information relating to her/his probable post-operative experience in order to decrease her/his pre-operative anxiety and post-operative pain, I am using interpersonal skills. Similarly, if I encourage a disoriented man to drink his tea, I am using interpersonal skills. Finally, if I help a student to understand the meaning of 'iatrogenesis', I am using interpersonal skills. These skills are also used in all areas of nursing management, interdisciplinary team-work, and in ordinary day-to-day contact with friends, family, colleagues and people generally.

Because it is impossible for two or more people to function in a collaborative way without the use of interpersonal skills, these skills are universally used in all types of nursing activity. That they are monopolised by, or more central to, areas such as psychiatric nursing for example, is an unfortunate myth which has done much to prevent their universal recognition in nursing.

Types of Interpersonal Skill Use

Interpersonal skills can be used to reach three major types of goal: *direct goal (formal)*; *direct goal (informal)*; and *indirect goal*.

Direct Goal (Formal) (Example: one-to-one psychotherapy designed to improve patient's assertiveness)

Here, specific and pre-determined goals which are usually known to both parties are pursued. Regular and planned contact, usually in the privacy of a consulting room or office, takes place. This contact, which typically consists of an hour-long meeting at the same time each day, may well be the only contact between patient and therapist. The therapist may be a nurse or, more frequently, a medical or para-medical professional such as a clinical psychologist. The contribution which staff other than the therapist make to the patient's on-going therapy is usually regarded as relatively unimportant. Indeed, it may be actively discouraged. Another form which *direct goal (formal)* interpersonal skill use may take is the sociotherapeutic approach, with the use of group therapy (rather than the one-to-one) being the focus of this treatment format. The *direct goal (formal)* is one which has been identified and chosen by one or both of the participants. It is relatively structured, formal, perhaps documented, may be reliant on interpersonal skills theory, and is reflected in the organisation and recognition of a 'client-therapist' relationship.

This use of this type of interpersonal skill in nursing is not a natural outcome of developments within the profession. Rather, it is a relatively foreign use which has been 'borrowed' from (occasionally imposed by) other professional groups who had developed, or were developing, sociotherapeutic or psychotherapeutic approaches. Although this new and increasingly employed use of interpersonal skill in a structured, formal and goal-directed fashion is *not* a natural outgrowth of nursing practice, it is regarded by many as a legitimate part of the nursing role, an assumption which requires considerable examination and challenge on various counts.

First, this formal use of interpersonal skills, as used in the practice of psychotherapy for example, has been developed, tested, researched and evaluated in an environment which is radically different to that in which most nurses work. This approach has been developed and used by those (non-nurses) who have relatively short term, structured contact with patients. The doctors or psychologists who may see the patient, or patient group, for one hour daily are the common examples of this approach.

Second, very little existing interpersonal skill theory, of the *direct goal* type, takes account of how a continuing interpersonal relationship/contact should be used. Although the nursing literature is taking more account of the fact that nurse-patient contact is over a 24 hour period in many instances, much confusion continues to exist. In one ward I visited recently, run as a therapeutic community, the nursing contribution to formal *direct goal* therapy was expected to last for one hour per day.

Third, many nurses and other health care professionals do not (rightly or wrongly) see this as a legitimate part of the nurses' role. Nurses may be perceived, and see themselves, as lacking the appropriate training for this role. Despite the fact that many other health care professionals have no training in this subject, nurses continue to see the use of *direct goal (formal)* interpersonal skill as being 'their' job (that is, the 'job' of non-nurse health care professionals).

The classic example of a *direct goal (formal)* approach might be the daily one-to-one, or group, meeting in which the client and therapist meet in order that the therapist can help the client come to terms with, or get rid of, an intrapersonal or interpersonal problem. Examples of such problems might be a husband-wife conflict, a fear of meeting people, or a pathological fear of gaining weight. Further examples might be an unrealistic reluctance to exercise following a coronary thrombosis, an inability to accept the disfiguring effects of surgery, or an overdependence on others during, or following, any illness.

The solutions to these, and a multitude of other similar problems, are long term. They undoubtedly require intensive, structured and carefully planned use of interpersonal skills which should be consistently used by all those who come into contact with the client. Clearly, if the client is an in-patient, and in close contact with nurses on an hour-to-hour basis, the nurses are in a potentially unique position in which to provide this type of care, *should they wish to do so.*

Direct Goal (Informal) (Example: encouraging a patient to 'help around the ward')

Here, rather more general, and sometimes vague, goals are pursued; these may or may not be known to all those involved. For example, goals may have been set for a patient who may be unaware of them. Alternatively, the patient may be aware of the goals which have been made known to *some* of the staff. The structure and content of the patient-staff contact is usually relatively informal and unplanned. Indeed, the patient and some staff members may regard participation as optional. The use of this type of interpersonal skill can, theoretically, extend to all the patient's waking hours. The staff most commonly involved in this approach are ward-based nursing staff, with others such as medical and para-medical staff rarely being involved. The general emphasis in *direct goal (informal)* use of interpersonal skills use is on informality, an experiential approach and a heavy commitment by nursing staff.

This approach may be used to deal with the same sort of problems as are dealt with by use of the *direct goal (formal)* approach. Thus, the goals may be the same; the difference lies in the means of achieving these goals. Because this (relatively unstructured and informal) use of interpersonal skills in nursing does not comply with the 'definition' of the formal and structured interventions used in the established 'therapeutic' approaches to patient care, it may be discounted as a 'legitimate' form of therapy. Consequently, interpersonal skills used by nurses may be (wrongly) perceived by nurses and researchers as either not being used, or infrequently used. I contend that these researchers, many of whom have been nurses, may apply the wrong criteria *(direct goal, formal)* when they look for interpersonal skills usage in nursing. Part of the reason for this may well be that these investigators have received their research training in the behavioural sciences, and may not readily adapt suitable paradigms to the nursing context. I also propose that a very different conclusion may be reached if the *direct goal (informal)* criteria are applied.

The *direct goal (informal)* is one which has been identified in a rather more general and diffuse way, relative to the *direct goal (formal)* approach. It is largely unstructured, informal, probably not documented, and may be reliant on experiential 'training' rather than on a formal training. It does not depend on the existence of a recognised client-therapist relationship, rather it is an approach which (potentially) involves all who come into contact with the client. Staff who wish to help the patient move towards a particular goal can do so, those who wish to 'opt out' can do so.

This use of interpersonal skills in nursing is a natural and well established development within nursing generally. It is an approach which is neither borrowed from, nor imposed by, other professional groups. The unique feature of this approach is that it is built into the normal, day-to-day contact between nurses and patients. It relies on the use of real and natural experience which both parties encounter in the time they spend together. Of course, the 'normality' of these experiences is relative, in that a nurse-patient environment and relationship exists. However, it is much more 'normal' than, for example, the one-to-one, or group, interaction and/or relationship which are used to facilitiate the *direct goal (formal)* approach.

Indirect Goal (Example: preparing a patient for medical treatment such as electro-convulsive therapy)

Here, the nurse responds to the requirements of other health care professionals and acts as an intermediary between them and the patient. The nurse acts as a facilitator, as a means by which others may reach their goals. Nurse-patient contact, and the use of interpersonal skills, in this *indirect goal* manner, are recognised as integral and important parts of the nurses' role (they are not optional). Some years ago during a visit which I was making to a number of acute admission wards (almost all of which were locked) in hospitals in the USA, I was asked 'How do you manage to nurse patients in *unlocked* acute admission wards in Scotland?' On reflection, the answer to this question must have much to do with the use of *indirect goal* interpersonal skills. It is my firm view that the use of informal, experiential and unstructured interpersonal skills by nurses plays an important part in causing patients to accept and participate in the treatment carried out by other professionals. A large part of the work of the nurse is to assist other professionals, medical staff and physiotherapists for example, to reach the specific goals which they are trying to reach. This traditional and well established role, in which the nurse is a *facilitator*, is essential to the successful functioning of many (if not all) other professionals who work in a hospital context.

The use of interpersonal skills to reach *indirect goals* (those which have been selected by others) is usually informal and unstructured.

Examples of this type of interpersonal skill use might be: persuading a reluctant patient to take prescribed medications; assisting an anxious patient to cope with submitting to surgery; teaching a diabetic patient how to determine the required dose of insulin; and enabling a paranoid person to talk about her/his delusions, thus enabling a psychiatrist to make a diagnosis and/or prescribe appropriate treatment.

Interpersonal Skills Use in Nursing

Any discussion of interpersonal skills use in nursing must take account of the existence of diverse types of interpersonal skills usage. Indeed, it might be argued that the use of such skills is both a myth *and* a reality, depending on which type is being considered.

It has become fashionable in recent years to criticise the extent to which nurses fail to make use of interpersonal skills (this criticism has been particularly strong when made by nurses generally, and nurse researchers in particular). My view is that, rather than apply the concept, definition and criteria of interpersonal skills use which belong to non-nurses, we should make a fresh examination of those interpersonal skills that we *do* use. My prediction is that such an examination would add a new dimension to our understanding of interpersonal skills use in a health care setting.

Interpersonal Skills Use in Nursing: The Myth

There is little doubt that the use of interpersonal skills in nursing, in the *formal* and *structured* sense is minimal. Whereas medical and para-medical staff, such as clinical psychologists and social workers, are increasingly making use of a structured and formal approach to inter-personal skill use, it is (unfortunately) rather unusual for nurses to do so. This point applies equally to psychiatric and non-psychiatric health care settings.

The myth, therefore, applies to *one* type of interpersonal skills use; the *direct goal (formal)* approach. The myth only applies to the formal and structured approaches which have been developed and used by non-nurses in order to meet the requirements of their relatively restric-ted access to patients. The existence of this 'myth' should be seen more as a reluctance of nurses to use this approach, rather than as an innate (or learned) inability. It is the experience of a number of nurse clinicians and teachers that a high level of psychotherapeutic skill can be achieved by nurses who wish to use interpersonal skills in a formal and structured manner.

Interpersonal Skills Use in Nursing: The Reality

That nurses make use of interpersonal skills is not a myth, it is a reality. The reason it is often (wrongly) perceived as a myth are manifold. First, a relatively narrow definition has been applied. This has been developed for a non-nursing purpose, and is unable to identify and describe the use of these skills in nursing. Second, the nature and complexity of nursing are poorly understood, not least by nurses themselves. Third, nurses are often reluctant to describe their work as being anything other than 'routine', 'basic', 'ordinary' or 'just common sense'. The result of this underselling and undervaluing of the nurses' contribution, is that much of their actual and potential positive contribution to health care (including that which depends on interpersonal skills use) will fail to be formally identified. Fourth, the use of these skills in a structured and formal way brings with it an added responsibility and accountability which nurses are only just beginning to accept.

Despite the circumstances which combine to minimise the apparent lack of interpersonal skills use in nursing, the reality is that these skills are fundamental to, and pervade, the practice of nursing. The task of nursing is to identify, analyse, describe, utilise and capitalise on these skills, which are used by nurses, in a way which is unique. This uniqueness, and its importance to the success of the provision of health care is demonstrated in an anecdote which was related to me by a young man who had to be hospitalised for medical treatment of an eye ailment. The impatience of the man during this, his first, hospitalisation, coupled with a natural shyness and feeling of inferiority, resulted in considerable anxiety and reluctance to stay for the duration of his treatment. When I asked why he did stay and complete the treatment, he replied; 'It was because of the nurses. They made me feel welcome, they made me feel at home. After a while, they made me feel just like one of them, they made me want to stay and finish the treatment.' This and many other examples of interpersonal skills use in nursing have developed in an experiential way over the years. It would be a great pity if we allowed our familiarity with these skills to cause us to ignore their existence and importance.

The Future

I propose that nurses in *all* specialities must make an urgent examination of the manner in which they make use of interpersonal skills, and of the manner in which they might make *further* use of them. Such an examination, which would include theoretical and applied perspectives, would enable appropriate educational strategies to be developed which would complement the existing experiential opportunities which exist in clinical settings. The uniqueness of the way in which nurses use interpersonal skills demands that *they* develop an appropriate educational input which is designed to prepare nurses to fill their role. Because of the wealth of experience that nurses have in using interpersonal skills in a way which cannot be matched by any other professional group, and because of the availability of theoretical perspectives which have been developed by other professional groups, we are now in a position to recognise and formalise these skills, *should we wish to do so*. It is my view that the most productive use of interpersonal skills in nursing is a multi-directional approach, in which *direct goal (formal), direct goal (informal) and indirect goal* approaches are used.

References

Cormack, D.F.S. (1983) *Psychiatric Nursing Described*, Churchill Livingstone: Edinburgh

General Nursing Council (1982) 'Training Syllabus: Register of Nurses, Mental Nursing', General Nursing Council for England and Wales: London.

8 DEFICIENCIES IN KEY INTERPERSONAL SKILLS

Peter Maguire

Introduction

The quality of nurse-patient communication is fundamental to good nursing care. Many nurses, however, reveal a level of interpersonal skill that militates against their patients' chances of receiving the most effective nursing care. I will draw on my work with general, psychiatric and specialist nurses to give examples of key deficiencies and illustrate more 'skilled' ways of handling situations. By doing this, I hope that nurses and nurse tutors will be able to recognise common problems and help each other and their students to overcome them. The examples I use are drawn from recordings of nurses talking to patients in a variety of settings.

Key Communication Tasks

To be fully effective, all nurses must be able to communicate with patients in a way which promotes trust and encourages them to disclose all relevant problems. If problems are identified incorrectly, the plan of care will be inappropriate to the patient's needs and may lead to a wasting of both time and resources. Once the problems have been identified, nurses have to offer some explanation of what is wrong. They should do this by establishing both what the patient already knows and what the patient now wishes to know. They can then tailor their information to the needs of the individual patient, instead of hiding behind outmoded rules of telling or not telling. Unnecessary worry and misunderstandings should then be avoided.

It is also important to explain any treatment or procedures in such a way that patients fully grasp what is planned, and are also given the reasons if they wish to know them. However well problems and treatments are explained, their very nature may provoke distress and worry. So, how patients feel about what they have been told should be explored before any reassurance or further explanation is attempted. If this is not done, reassurance may be misplaced and ineffective. Nurses should check that patients fully understand the doctors' treatment plans as well

116

as any nursing procedures. They will then be in a position to correct any misconceptions or fears and reinforce advice. Otherwise, patients may fail to comply with advice and stop the treatment.

Many illnesses and their treatments cause substantial practical, social and psychological problems. These can intensify suffering, impair day-to-day functioning and cause tension within the family unless they are recognised and dealt with. They will only be detected if nurses involved in aftercare monitor the patients' physical, social and psychological adjustment.

As well as these basic communication tasks, there are some more difficult situations which nurses have to try and handle.

Difficult Situations

The Angry Patient. Nurses may be faced with a furious patient or relative complaining about medical or nursing neglect or negligence. Unless they know how to defuse the situation and help the patient or relative express or explore these angry feelings, serious problems can result. In addition to personal distress, the patient may even sue the hospital.

The Withdrawn Patient. On a busy ward, patients who are withdrawn and uncommunicative can cause anger and frustration because they may come to be regarded as difficult and uncooperative. Such attitudes will only increase patients' withdrawal. However, nurses who have a knowledge of why patients become withdrawn, and the skills required to draw the patient out, can favourably affect the situation.

The Dying Patient. If patients are to have an opportunity of dying peacefully, they need to be able to discuss any practical, social or psychological concerns that are worrying them. If dialogue is avoided or blocked because the nurses do not feel equipped to deal with difficult questions that might arise, the patients are likely to become more anxious and depressed. This will then reduce the threshold at which physical symptoms like pain are experienced. Pain control is made more difficult and patients may become withdrawn. Consequently, important areas of unfinished business (like a man telling his partner how much he loved and valued her) will not be dealt with and he may die a stormy death. His partner will then be much less likely to resolve her grief and may even use an unhelpful means of tranquillising her suffering, like alcohol, or develop agoraphobia or depressive illness.

Upset/Bereaved Relatives. Nurses are often in the position of having to summon a relative to hospital in order to break bad news, for example, 'There's been a marked deterioration in her condition I'm afraid', or 'I'm afraid I've got bad news for you'. Unless such news is broken in a certain way, it may cause problems later. The relative may feel that something went wrong and that the hospital is concealing this.

Deficiencies in Key Skills

Since these communication tasks are central to good nursing care, it should be expected that all nurses possess the relevant skills. Sadly, it has been firmly established that, like doctors (Fletcher, 1980), this is not the case. (Jill Macleod Clark, Chapter 1, reviews the development of research relating to this issue.) Tape recordings of nurses talking with real patients on wards, within clinics or patients' homes, with simulated patients, or in role-play have revealed a consistent pattern of deficiencies in the relevant communication skills. Contrary to expectation, these are not remedied by experience. I will now consider some of these common deficiencies in key skills, as portrayed in the recordings of nurse-patient conversations.

The Identification of Problems

In a follow-up study of women undergoing mastectomy for breast cancer, the nurses were able to recognise only 20 per cent of those women who had developed an anxiety state, depressive illness or body image problems (Maguire *et al.*, 1980). This poor detection of psychosocial morbidity represents a widespread problem within nursing and medicine, and is due to several factors, including nursing priorities and lack of assessment skills.

Nursing Priorities. In nursing, the emphasis is usually on physical illness and practical aspects of care. Talking with patients is perceived as less important and less effective. Nurses who like to spend time talking with patients can find themselves criticised for not 'pulling their weight' with practical tasks. (See Chapter 4 by Ann Faulkner for further discussion of organisational constraints on nurses wishing to talk more with patients.)

Patient Assessment. This focus on physical problems is reflected in the content of most assessments. There will be a clear account of the major physical signs and symptoms but little if any coverage of how patients feel about the illness or its impact on their work, personal relationships, sex lives, mood or plans for the future. Thus an experienced stoma nurse produced the following assessment:

> Mrs T is a 54 year old married woman with three grown-up children. She had a colostomy for rectal cancer four months ago. She called in at the clinic to see me because she was having trouble with her bag. It had been leaking and causing an offensive smell. She had stopped going out much because of it. Otherwise she appears to be coping well. I've given her a new bag and will call on her in a week's time to see how she is getting on.

Independent assessment of the patient revealed a different picture. The woman had indeed been having problems with smell and leakage, but there were other reasons why she asked for help. She had serious sexual problems even though her general relationship was 'reasonable'. She had become very depressed to the point of feeling life was hopeless unless all these difficulties could be resolved. She had begun to sleep badly and found everything an effort. She felt she was an increasing burden and no longer of value as a person or a woman.

The stoma nurse was asked to do an assessment on another patient and this was tape-recorded. This revealed a common pattern of deficiencies that nurses display in talking to patients, which reduces the value of their time spent together.

Specific Skill Deficiencies

In this section, I will illustrate the specific skill deficiencies, with reference to the stoma nurse's assessment of her second patient.

Lack of Structure. Although the nurse was meeting the patient for the first time, she failed to make her role explicit. She merely said, 'I'm here to see if you have been having any problems with your stoma.' This made the patient feel (wrongly) that the nurse was solely interested in her bag, and not in her as a person. The nurse did not indicate how much time she had to spend. So the patient felt that there would not be enough time to deal with her worries about recurrence and spread of her cancer, and strong feelings of stigma and lack of worth. As the interview progressed, the nurse focused on the illness and bag before asking general questions like 'Are your family all right?' Her agenda did not include how the patient had felt about her illness and stoma. Nor did it include any enquiry about how her relationships had been affected, particularly her relationship with her husband and their sex life. No questions were asked about daily functioning except how she was managing her chores. The possibility that symptoms of anxiety and depression might be present was not considered although the patient was excessively worried about recurrence.

After the general questions about the family had revealed little, the nurse closed the interview without warning. She said 'Thank's a lot: I'm glad the bag's OK. I'd better be going. Get in touch if there are any problems.' Had she warned the patient 'I'm going to have to stop in a few minutes. So far you've said your stoma is working all right. Have there been any other problems?', the woman might have disclosed her true concerns. As it was, she was left feeling that the nurse was mainly concerned with her bag and that it was not legitimate for her to mention other matters.

Lack of Technique. The tape-recording exposed some clear problems of technique which also hindered disclosure of problems. These included:

(1) Faulty question style: the nurse used leading questions, which invited a particular answer, such as 'Your stoma's been working well, hasn't it?', instead of open questions which would generate more useful data, such as 'How has your stoma been?'. Similarly she said 'You've been going out all right?', instead of 'How much have you been out in the last week?'.

(2) Poor acknowledgement of cues: when the nurse began by asking 'Your stoma's been working well, hasn't it?', the patient said 'Well yes, I suppose it has, but I've been a bit worried sometimes . . .'. The nurse seized on the 'suppose it has' and rightly checked that the stoma and bag were all right. She failed to acknowledge the cue 'worried'. Had she said 'You said you were a bit worried . . .' and asked (negotiating) '. . . would you like to tell me about it?', the patient might have disclosed her concerns about stigma and recurrence immediately.

(3) Insufficient clarification; when the nurse asked 'How have your family been?', (a useful open question directing attention to the family), the patient replied 'Oh, they are all right — unlike me.' Hearing the '. . . unlike me . . .', the nurse assumed she was referring to her illness and colostomy. Had she clarified this cue by asking 'How do you mean — unlike me?', the strong feelings of stigma and

feelings of being of little value might have emerged.

(4) Problems with control: throughout this interview, the nurse was too controlling. She gave the patient little space to talk and often interrputed to pursue her line of enquiry. She clearly felt under pressure of time because of other patients who had to be seen that day. Sometimes nurses demonstrate the opposite difficulty. They allow patients to talk at length about matters unrelated to the task in hand. They do so because they hope the patient will eventually return to the subject. Yet, in reality, the patient rarely does. Unless they know how to interrupt and bring the patient back to the point, much time will be wasted. An example of how this might be done is as follows: 'You've been telling me about your first heart attack and that's helpful — but would you mind if I first concentrated on this last attack?'.

(5) Needless repetition: although nurses, like doctors, commonly complain that there is insufficient time to assess patients properly, much time is wasted through needless repetition. In this interview, the nurse covered the stoma and bag three times as if to reassure herself she had covered an important area adequately. She was not helped by her reluctance to take notes. Had she covered these aspects fully, just once, she would have saved much time.

In addition to those specific skills outlined above, nurses also lack more general communication skills.

General Skill Deficiencies

General deficiencies in skill, in the context of patient assessment, can lead to inappropriate nursing care plans, which can in turn affect recovery.

Lack of Precision. Plans of care depend on how a patient's problems are formulated and understood. For example, a man with severe and painful rheumatoid arthritis was assessed on admission to a medical ward and the assessment tape-recorded. He was judged to be severely handicapped and to have become depressed because of this and the pain. It was decided that his 'depression' would recover as his arthritis responded to treatment. Instead, he got progressively more depressed and difficult to manage. Subsequent assessment revealed why he was so depressed. His depression had begun two years previously, following his wife's death from cancer. He could not accept her death or the resultant loneliness. The latest attack of painful arthritis was the final straw. A revised care plan included treatment of the depressive illness and grief therapy. He made a full recovery. Had the nurse who carried out the original assessment not merely accepted the patient's claim 'I've got like this because of the arthritis,' but checked 'When exactly did these depressed feelings start?', she could have uncovered the real cause.

Lack of Clarification of Jargon. A patient was admitted to a psychiatric ward, and he was assessed by a staff nurse. He claimed to be 'confused', and the nurse proceeded to ask questions suggestive of an organic confusional state. Thus, she checked about the patient's orientation to time, place and date. Only belatedly did she realise that the patient had used 'confused' to indicate he was perplexed by hearing voices and worried that there was a plot to kill him. She had mistakenly assumed he was using appropriate jargon.

Lack of Appropriate Style of Questioning. The use of leading questions was mentioned above. Sometimes nurses fail to get adequate data because they ask several questions at once, and the patient responds to only one element, as for example, 'Now you say you've had a pain in your stomach. Is it worse when you eat? How bad is it? Does anything relieve it?'. Because of the complexity of the questioning, the patient would not know which part to answer first, and consequently may omit valuable information.

Lack of Response to Non-Verbal Cues. Patients often given non-verbal cues about their problems. Through tone of voice, posture, facial expression or emotion, they may indicate that they are worried, sad, angry or perplexed. It is rare for nurses to acknowledge this by saying, for example, 'When you mentioned your children, you looked upset: would you like to talk about it?'. If they were to make such observations, they might well encourage patients to discuss concerns they find too difficult to raise themselves. In some nursing settings, the use of non-verbal cues in assessing patient needs becomes even more critical (see, for example Pat Ashworth's discussion of interpersonal skills in intensive care settings, Chapter 10).

Inadequate Provision of Information. When nurses respond to patients' needs for information, they tend to give it inadequately. Frequently, too much information is given at once, and it is rare for checks that the patient has understood to be made. The order and importance of the information is not taken into account, and consequently data about diagnosis, treatment, adverse effects and prognosis may be intermingled. Patients are then unlikely to recall, accurately, what they are told. In addition, they may be left with serious misapprehensions: 'She told me I must rest. I thought she meant complete rest. When I went to the clinic, the doctor told me off for not exercising enough. I was so furious. I didn't realise that not exercising would make my joints worse.' Nurses, like doctors, tend to give information prematurely: that is, before they have properly established patients' knowledge and concerns. For example,

> *Nurse*: 'There's no need to worry about this operation. They will take the lump away and examine it under a microscope. If it is serious, they will probably decide to take your breast away to make sure it is all removed.'
> *Patient*: 'That's all very well. That's exactly what my sister was told. She was dead within six months.' Had the nurse realised how the patient felt, she might have proceeded as follows: 'I realise you were shattered by your sister's death, and I'm glad you told me about it. But I've checked with the hospital. Her cancer was different. It was at a much later stage. That's probably why treatment failed.'

Bryn Davis (Chapter 9) gives a comprehensive review of studies of preoperative information giving by nurses.

Nurses may feel handicapped by rules laid down by doctors, and avoid telling patients much about their illness or treatment. There is, though, a way out of this. When asked 'Have I got cancer?', they can reflect the question back by saying 'I'd be happy to answer, but first I would like to know just why you are asking now.' The patient will then usually indicate that s/he realises that s/he may have cancer because s/he has continued to lose weight despite treatment. The nurse has a choice. S/he can lie and say 'Don't be silly: of course it's not cancer': pass the buck by saying 'I don't know, you'd better ask the doctor'; or honestly say 'Yes, I'm afraid it is cancer, *but* but we should still be able to do something about it.' Most patients will find this last reply more helpful than the others.

Inadequate Provision of Reassurance. One alternative open to the nurse in answering patients' (difficult) questions, is to give reassurance. As with information, reassurance is only effective when nurses first establish what the patient is concerned about and why. In practice, this happens only occasionally. Instead, nurses tend to offer reassurance prematurely, as for example:

Nurse: 'Of course you're worried. There's no need to be. Everything will be all right'.
Patient: 'That's what they told my mother when she had her chest pains, and look what happened to her.'
Nurse: 'How do you mean?'
Patient: 'They put a tube into her lung to see what was happening. They initially said it was all right, but it proved to be cancer.'

Had the nurse established this fact first, she could have tailored her attempts at reassurance accordingly. 'In view of what happened to your mother you are bound to be worried. But we are pretty confident your pain is due to an infection and not cancer.'

Some nurses try to reduce patients' worries by offering *false reassurance*. Thus, they claim there will be no problems, even when this is not likely to be the case. They do so in the belief that this will help patients cope, and facilitates adjustment. An example might be a nurse talking to a woman about to undergo a mastectomy: 'There's no need to worry. We have very good prostheses these days. I'm sure we can find one to suit you. I'm sure this will help you.' In reality, at least one in five mastectomy patients will develop body image problems, despite being helped to obtain breast prostheses. The nurse should, perhaps, have said: 'I can see you have been worrying about losing a breast. I'll do my best to help you find a prosthesis to suit you. That should help. If it doesn't, you must tell me. I should then be able to do something about it.' (Mastectomy nursing raises some critical issues for the effective deployment of interpersonal skills, and these are discussed by Ann Tait in Chapter 11.)

When patients admit they have been distressed by a diagnosis or treatment, there is considerable risk that the nurse will dismiss it as normal, and so block further discussion that could have been beneficial. How often can the following, or something like it, be heard in the name of reassurance? 'Of course you are upset: everybody is at this stage. You'll soon settle down.'

Lack of Ability to Handle Difficult Situations.

(1) *Angry/withdrawn patients*: When handling angry or withdrawn patients, there is often a marked reluctance to confront the situation by saying something like, 'You sound very angry. Would you like to tell me

why?' or 'I can see you are finding it hard to talk to me. What's making it so difficult?' Instead, nurses get into a verbal (sometimes physical) 'battle' with their patients.

(2) *The dying patient*: Relatively few nurses appear to have the confidence and skills required if they are to enter into an effective dialogue with dying patients. They tend to restrict their attention to symptom control because this is 'safer'. When patients try to discuss crucial issues, they tend to use 'distancing tactics', including ignoring cues, giving false or premature reassurance, switching the topic, and so on. Ultimately, they may pass the buck by saying 'You should discuss this with the doctor.' Nurses' deficiencies here frequently lead to increased patient distress at a time when they most need understanding and realistic support. (Peter Banister and Carolyn Kagan, Chapter 3, address some of the issues surrounding the use of interpersonal skills with dying patients.)

Upset/Bereaved Relatives.

Similarly, nurses feel uneasy and uncertain when faced with bereaved, angry or upset relatives. They do not usually confront the central emotion — 'You look upset', 'You seem very angry' — or follow this acknowledgement by saying,' Would you like to tell me about it? Instead, they often become defensive — 'That's not fair, we did all we could', or even angry themselves — 'You've no right to say that.' So, rather than alleviating distress and anger, they often intensify it.

From the above discussion, we can see that both specific and general interpersonal skill deficiencies are common in a number of nursing settings. I will now discuss, briefly, some of the reasons for such deficiencies.

Why Are Nurses Deficient in Key Interpersonal Skills?

Several of the contributors to this volume offer some explanation as to why nurses may not always display effective interpersonal skills. I believe the crucial factors to be related to the (lack of) training that nurses receive.

Inappropriate Models

It is generally assumed that nurses learn the relevant communication skills through their ordinary training and experience. This assumption rests on the belief that experienced nurses afford appropriate models. Yet, how can they, if they, themselves, have not participated in the relevant skills training? Indeed, what is clear is that the models given to nurses have been deficient in two respects. First, the areas to be covered have not been adequately explained, even within the nursing process. Second, little attempt has been made to make the relevant skills explicit by use of printed handouts and videotaped interviews, for example.

Reliance on Indirect Methods of Assessing Communication Skills

Like medical training, few nurses are observed while interviewing their patients or relating to relatives. Consequently, their communication skills are judged indirectly on the basis of what their colleagues and patients say about them. Yet this can give a misleading impression of their real level of skill, and deficiencies will remain unnoticed.

Neglect in Training

As several other contributors have pointed out, there is a dearth of interpersonal skills training in nurse education (see Part V for advances in this field). Thus, even if appropriate models of interviewing are taught, feedback of performance given by means of audio/videotape, and the opportunity to practise skills is afforded, this may take up only a minor part of training, because it is given low priority. Students may then question its value.

How Can Nurses Improve Their Interpersonal Skills?

There are many different approaches to the teaching and learning of interpersonal skills generally, and in nursing specifically (see Part V). In the training of doctors, the teaching of essential interviewing skills has proved effective when it includes practice, followed by audio or television replay and discussion (Maguire, 1984). Importantly, these skills are still evident four to six years after training (Maguire, Fairburn and Fletcher, 1985). When acquired by nurses through similar training, they have led to a major reduction in the level of patients' psychological and social morbidity (Maguire *et al.*, 1980, 1983). Thus, it is likely that if such training were included in general training, great benefits to patients and relatives would follow. To be truly effective, training would have to acknowledge that 'tuning in' to how patients and relatives have adapted to illness can bring nurses close to suffering, and this exacts an emotional price. Methods of coping — even survival in the profession — will therefore also need to be considered. These might include the use of support groups, regular time out, or rationing the number of difficult situations that are encountered.

It is clear, though, that despite these considerations, the deficiencies in interpersonal skills use amongst nurses are great enough, and important enough to patient care, to warrant immediate attention. It is only when interpersonal skills training is given high priority in nurse education that patients will receive the most effective nursing care.

References

Fletcher, C. (1980) 'Listening and Talking to Patients', *British Medical Journal, 281*, 931-3

Maguire, P. (1984) 'Communication Skills and Patient Care' in A. Steptoe and A. Mathews (eds), *Health Care and Human Behaviour*, Academic Press : London

Maguire, P., Tait, A., Brooke, M., Thomas, C. and Sellwood, R. (1980) 'The Effect of Counselling on the Psychiatric Morbidity Associated With Mastectomy', *British Medical Journal, 2*, 1454-6

Maguire, P., Tait, A., Brooke, M., Thomas, C., and Sellwood, R. (1983) 'The Effect of Counselling on Physical Disability and Social Recovery After Mastectomy', *Clinical Oncology, 9*, 319-24

Maguire, P., Fairburn, S., and Fletcher, C. (1985) 'Doctors Talking to Patients (1): The effects of interview training are still evident 3 to 5 years later', in preparation

9 THE CLINICAL EFFECT OF INTERPERSONAL SKILLS: THE IMPLEMENTATION OF PRE-OPERATIVE INFORMATION GIVING

Bryn Davis

Introduction

The concerns of this chapter are twofold. First, there is a concern with the role of the nurse as communicator and, second, there is a concern with the implementation of research findings, particularly in the clinical field. Together, these concerns gain expression in the impressive influence on patient care in general and post-operative patient progress in particular by nurses fulfilling their communications role.

When asked who should give pre-operative information to patients, doctors, nurses and physiotherapists on a surgical unit indicated that the primary source should be the trained nurse, and the next should be the senior house-officer/registrar (Davis, 1983). Some differences of opinion were expressed as to who should give which items of information, but the main point of interest here was the major role in patient communication allocated to trained nurses by two groups of their professional colleagues. Much evidence exists, also, showing that the patients, themselves, see the nurse as the person from whom to gain information (Cartwright, 1964; Carstairs, 1970; Raphael, 1977; The Royal Commission, 1978). Not only do patients want information from nurses, but there is increasing evidence that such information is beneficial to the patients' post-operative progress (see literature review in the next section).

However, acknowledging the importance of nurse-patient communication in general, and with respect to post-operative information in particular, one must still ask the question 'can nurses, as part of their everyday care of patients, achieve the same benefits from communication as the researchers have in their controlled and specially supervised settings?' The question of the implementation of research into nursing practice is one that is a major cause for concern wherever nursing research is undertaken. Although projects concerning nursing practice are in a minority (Lelean, 1982), even those that are carried out have, it seems, little chance of being utilised. (A similar issue, of extending a 'specialist nurse' research project to the ward nurse situation, is explored by Ann Tait in Chapter 11, with reference to mastectomy nursing.)

In the United States, extensive programmes have been introduced in attempts to study the process of implementation (Horsley, Crane and Bingle, 1978; Krueger, Nelson and Nolanin, 1978), and there have been similar efforts reported in the United Kingdom (Towell and Harries, 1979). The question has also been considered of major importance in Continental Europe (Grypdonck *et al.*, 1979). As Lelean (1982) points out, the essential factor in successful implementation is the bringing together of researchers, managers, educators and practitioners as a team, to initiate and pursue policies of planned change.

Hunt (1981), has identified five factors that may explain why the implementation of research is so limited. These anticipate the four offered by Lelean (1982). The two sets involve making the findings available and accessible; assessing their relevance and usability; and making use of them (for a further discussion of this, see Peter Banister and Carolyn Kagan's Chapter 3). These different aspects indicate the importance of including researchers, managers and educators in any attempt to introduce research findings into practice. As Hunt (1981) suggests, in some instances, some practitioners are not allowed to innovate. Managers with the necessary authority and support for the attempt have a vital role to play. The preparation of staff in the new techniques or procedures is necessary if the innovation is to be supported by the informed participation of the whole nursing team. Lelean (1982), in her discussion, also pinpointed the importance of helping the practitioners, educators and managers to comprehend the full import of particular research reports. Researchers who can readily communicate their work to colleagues are a great asset to any innovation programme.

One of the functions of this chapter is to try to make research findings available and, hopefully, comprehensible and applicable to nurses. The next section offers a literature review, discussing nursing research reports in the field of pre-operative information giving. This will be followed by a continuation of the discussion — *can nurses utilise research findings, and can they achieve the same kind of benefits*? The literature review covers four main issues involved in the topic of pre-operative information giving by nurses: the study of stress and, in particular, pain and anxiety; the role of information giving in stress reduction; the problems inherent in the definition of outcomes against which to evaluate the information-giving intervention; and the kinds of outcomes that have been demonstrated to be amenable to influence in this way.

Stress

Pre-operative preparation of patients has been a subject of concern for some time. In particular, the relation between stress and post-operative outcomes has been a topic of much debate. Most of the research done in this area has been related to a model of stress reduction, with stress being seen, as defined by Selye (1956), as *the state manifested by a specific syndrome which consists of all the non-specifically induced changes within a biological system.* Hayward (1975), Boore (1978) and Wilson-Barnett (1978) have all reviewed the literature in this area, and the following discussion has been much influenced by them.

Stress has, then, been defined as a physiological phenomenon with psychological links (Selye, 1956), and as being caused by environmental conditions, trauma, disease or emotional states. An alarm reaction was described by him, which is followed by the General Adaptation Syndrome, and which leads eventually, if the stress is not effectively relieved, to morbidity and perhaps death. This process involves biochemical changes and, in particular, adreno-cortical activity, which facilitates or creates the body's adaptation, or if in excess or prolonged, causes breakdown of normal tissue function. Some workers have emphasised the importance of psychological aspects; for example, Janis (1958) and Lazarus (1971), who claim that these are different from and not necessarily related to physiological stress. Psychological stress is related to uncertainty, loss of control, isolation, pain and a general sense of threat. Lazarus (1966) identified four major reactions to stress, two of which are psychological — the emotional and cognitive reactions related to the individual's interpretation of the situation; and two of which are physical — the psychomotor and physiological or hormonal.

Two main approaches to the study of stress can be identified in the literature. The first is a concern with the external threatening events that elicit the responses (Langer and Michaels, 1963) and the second is a concern with the reaction to stress in the individual. Discussions of the latter by Janis (1958) and Selye (1956) offer similar patterns or phases of response, including anticipation or alarm; adaptation by defence or escape; and deprivation, loss and possible morbidity. Stress can thus mean the stimulus (threatening event), the anticipation of this, the experience of it, or the long-term effects of the event. The importance of clear definition when discussing the issue has been emphasised by both Hayward (1975) and Boore (1978).

The relationship of stress to negative emotions, such as anxiety and depression, has been pointed out by Wilson-Barnett (1978). Anticipatory stress and the effectiveness or otherwise of adjustment of coping strategy can lead to anxiety; a sense of failure to cope, or loss, can lead to depression. It has also been recognised that anxiety can have an important function in facilitating performance by increasing the level of arousal (Hayward, 1975). Excessive arousal, however, leads to disruption of performance. Hayward also emphasised the importance of seeing anxiety both as a continuing trait or characteristic of the individual and as a learned state dependent on situational factors. This latter aspect of anxiety has been associated with endocrine activity (Speilberger, 1966), such as that indicated by Selye as being operative in stress reactions, and as described by Boore (1978) in her study of physiological manifestations of stress.

Pain has been described as both a stressor and a reaction to stress: as a stimulus and as experience. Attempts to study it in relation to stress phenomena are confounded by this problem. Hayward, in discussing this, described three theories of pain and considered these in the context of the relationship between stimulus and perception. Early workers tended to consider pain as a phenomenon involving specific receptors and nerve fibres, and specific centres in the brain. This approach has been criticised by Sternbach (1966), for example, who accepted the possibility of specific receptors and fibres but not necessarily the specificity of responses. Others have suggested that the perception of pain was related to particular patterns of nerve impulses along ordinary nerve fibres (for example, Weddell, 1962). A third theory involves a 'gate' mechanism in the dorsal spinal column, controlled by the central nervous system, which allows the inhibition of pain impulses from peripheral fibres and regulation of the flow of impulses to the brain (Melzack and Wall, 1965). In this way, it is argued, perception may be different from stimulus, and thus provide an explanation for the different experiences reported by individuals in response to similar or equally traumatic stimuli as described, for example, by Melzack and Torgerson (1971). Thus external factors influencing the nature of the stimulus and internal factors influencing the kind of perception of pain are important, but of particular importance are anxiety and coping strategies with respect to the latter.

Anxiety and pain have been the focus of research into the care of patients undergoing surgery and other invasive or threatening events. The importance of perception and other cognitive activities in coping with stress and in experiencing pain has offered an avenue for interventions to facilitate this coping. The reduction of uncertainty by giving information about the nature of the threatening event, and the experiences to be expected, and instructions in coping strategies such as exercises and methods of movement, are interventions therefore that theoretically could be applied to this end. The next part of this review considers some attempts to introduce procedures of this kind, the results of which are the focus of this study.

Outcomes

Table 9.1 shows post-operative outcomes that have been studied by nurses in relation to pre-operative preparation. The outcomes shown in the table are those amenable to observation and measurement by nurses. Other measures of a more specialist nature have been excluded. Psychological measures of anxiety and physiological measures of stress have been utilised in some studies and have shown significant differences between experimental and control groups (for example, Boore, 1978; Felton, Huss, Payne and Sersic, 1976; Hayward, 1975; Hegyvary and Chamings, 1975; Schmitt and Wooldridge, 1973). However, it is felt that the emphasis of future studies might be on patient outcomes related to the nursing role and within the range of nursing skills.

Outcomes are generally accepted as being alterations in health status. Zimmer (1974) uses the term 'patient health/wellness status'. Bloch (1975) also refers to health status but accepts (after Donabedian, 1970) that psychosocial, cognitive and behavioural factors should be included. She felt, however, that these should be termed 'intermediate outcomes'. This would suggest that the reduction of anxiety is an intermediate stage in, for example, the perception of pain by the patient, but not as a legitimate goal in itself. However, attempts to classify types of outcomes usually include a wider range than the physical implied by Bloch. Zimmer (1974), referring to outcomes as related to health status, also suggested that they were subject to change by nursing activities, whereas Hilger (1974) said that they were the end results of activities performed by the professionals. The difference between these two definitions illustrates one of the dilemmas facing attempts to

Table 9.1: Post-operative Outcomes, Related to the Nursing Role, Showing Significant Effects in Relation to Information Giving Non-significant Effects on the Right

Outcome Criteria						Studies						Non-significant
Doses analgesics		S	H	HC	FK	FF					V	B/LA/L
Pain experienced	L	S	H	HC		FF				J		B
Length of post-operative stay	DL	LA S	H	HC						J		FK/KT
Nausea and vomiting		S	H									S
Sleep		S	H	HC								H
Complications				HC			B					
Days to solid diet		S		HC								
Memory of operation			H					N				B
Mental state										J		B
Ventilation of lungs	LA				FK						KT	
Activities of daily living	LA				FK							
Ambulation		S								J		
Pulse rate		S					FF					
Blood pressure		S					FF					
Urine retention												
Physical wellbeing							FF					

Key

DL	Dumas et al. (1963)	FF	Flaherty et al. (1978)
LA	Lindeman et al. (1971)	N	Nolan (1977)
L	Luna (1971)	B	Boore (1978)
S	Schmitt et al. (1973)	J	Johnson et al. (1978)
H	Hayward (1975)	V	Voshall (1980)
HC	Hegyvary et al. (1975)	KT	King et al. (1982)
FK	Fortin et al. (1976)		

Source: *Nursing Times*, 77, April 2nd 1981.
Reproduced by kind permission of *Nursing Times*

evaluate nursing care and, in particular, to relate that evaluation to outcomes. As Bloch (1975) puts it, there should be patient care outcomes as the ideal, rather than nursing outcomes, medical outcomes or other outcomes. Her thesis here is that patient care is the function of the input of many interacting and cooperating professionals rather than professionals with isolated, discrete inputs.

Taylor (1974) assumes three points. First, that nursing care does affect the outcome of the patients' illnesses and has influence on their future health status. Secondly, that even though nursing shares responsibility for patient care with many health disciplines, there are outcomes that are primarily attributable to nursing care and these can be identified. Thirdly, there are also outcomes that are only partially or marginally attributable to nursing care and these, too, can be identified. McFarlane (1970) also criticised the outcome measures used in a series of American studies reviewed by her, on the grounds that they could not be demonstrated to be related solely to nursing activity.

Outcome Criteria

A major problem with the establishment of outcomes and with their relationship to nursing activities is that nursing procedures are not well defined; they vary from one setting to another and the consequences of even standard practices are not really known. Criterion measures of nursing care outcomes still need to be defined (Smith and Horn, 1973). This echoes an earlier call of Abdellah (1961), who defined a criterion measure as a score in the dependent variable to be predicted which can be used as an external basis for judgement to measure the effect of the stimuli applied to the experimental subjects. Abdellah also suggested that such criteria might be helpful in such situations as the effects of nursing practice on surgical patients' progress. Later, still pursuing the same theme, she argued that the lack of criterion measures in nursing puts a partial blindfold on nurses as they provide nursing care. She went on to say that criterion measures of nursing practice must derive from the dependent variables that indicate the effects of practice upon patient care (Abdellah and Levine, 1979). Here, dependent variable equates with nursing outcome as being specific to the patient population, but must be observable, qualifiable and useful (Aydelotte, 1973). Taylor (1974) adds that they must be stated as patient outcomes rather than nursing actions.

There does, however, seem to be a lack of clarity in the way in which such terms as 'criterion' have been used. Recently, Bloch (1975) has offered definitions of such terms. She defines criterion (or criterion variable, or parameter) as the value-free *name* of a variable believed or known to be a relevant indicator of the quality of patient care (medical care; nursing care). It must not be used as a *measure* of quantity or value. If we wish to obtain a measure of quantity or value, then we are dealing with a 'standard', which is defined as the desired and achievable level or range of performance. Bloch quotes Hagen (1972) as insisting that the term 'criterion' should never be used in the sense of a measure, score or value.

In Krumme's (1975) discussion of criterion referenced evaluation, she was arguing for criterion referenced evaluation as opposed to normative referenced evaluation. Popham and Husek (1969) also proposed, in their field, the establishment of criterion referenced measurements. They said that these were used to ascertain an individual's status with respect to some criterion, that is, a performance standard. They argued that they are devised to make decisions about individuals and treatments. Normative referenced assessment relates to an average performance for that population. The difference can, perhaps, be illustrated with an example. If a group of people are asked to perform some task and their performance is measured and scores obtained, then an acceptance of the top 25 per cent, whatever their scores, would be a norm referenced standard, whereas the acceptance of all those scoring over 75 per cent of the total possible score, for example, would be a criterion referenced standard.

There might be some conflict here with regard to the insistence of such as Aydelotte (1973) that outcome criteria must be specific to the patient population. However, it is possible to establish outcome criteria standards without reference to the norm of the patient population; outcome criteria and standards of performance in those criteria are related to an individual's needs rather than to the norm for that patient population. The relevance of these discussions to nursing practice has usually been with reference to the institution of individualised nursing care and the use of nursing care plans. This is the nub of Krumme's argument; and it is also relevant when attempting to evaluate at a more general level — at, say, ward, unit or hospital level. However, there is a use for normative referenced evaluation with either structural, process or outcome aspects of care. The choice between criterion referenced and normative referenced evaluation must depend on the purpose of the evaluation; whether the concern is to effect a comparison with others of a like sort, in terms of the criteria (normative referenced), or whether it is to effect an individual assessment in terms of the criteria alone (criteria referenced).

Post-operative Outcome Criteria

As can be seen in Table 9.1, a wide range of outcomes have been significantly influenced. However, it seems that some influences have been more readily replicated than others, and many have given rise to non-significant findings. Taking into account the number of non-significant and significant findings, it would seem that confident predictions of the influence of pre-operative information giving can be made with respect to 'doses of analgesics' and 'pain experienced', with marginally less confident predictions regarding 'length of post-operative stay'. Several outcomes were replicated and had no non-significant results, thus allowing confident predictions, namely: 'sleep', 'complications' and 'memory of operation'. Far less confident predictions can be made with respect to the other outcome measures, as the studies have revealed relatively higher numbers of non-significant findings.

The various studies listed in Table 9.1 also employed different methods of information giving and this also seems to be a factor in determining the effect on outcomes: most of the studies offered a mixture of sensory, procedural and coping information (Table 9.2). Three of the studies involved only instructions on coping strategies, breathing and movement exercises, and two a mixture of procedural information and coping strategies.

It is impossible to assess the relative effects of the different types of information in these studies, although Johnson *et al.* (1978) argue that it is possible to detect a more consistent effect from instructions about coping strategies. The design for their study did involve an evaluation of the differential effects of these three kinds of information. This design was influenced by the work of Langer *et al.* (1975) who differentially assessed information and a coping strategy. This was not a nursing study, however, and thus does not appear in the table; the information-giving was by psychologists. Johnson *et al.* argue, on the basis of other work concerning laboratory studies of threatening events (for example, Johnson, 1973; Johnson and Rice, 1974) and in clinical settings not involving surgery (for example, Johnson and Leventhal, 1974; Johnson, Kirchhoff and Endress, 1975; Johnson, Morrissey and Leventhal, 1973) that informational interventions that are relevant to the patient's point of view, and not based on nursing manuals or textbooks, are more consistent in facilitating coping with these threatening events. They suggest that a failure to provide this kind of information may explain the relatively inconsistent results for information giving in the nursing literature.

Table 9.2 Methods of Information Giving Used in the Various Studies Reviewed in the Pre-operative Information Giving Literature

Type	Researcher, Verbal	Researcher, Written/Taped	Nurses, Unstructured	Nurses, Structured
SPC	Luna (1971) Schmitt et al. (1973) Hayward (1975) Boore (1978) Voshall (1980)			Fortin et al. (1976)
PC	Dumas et al. (1963) Hegyvary et al. (1975)	Hegyvary et al. (1975)		
SC			Nolan (1977)	
C	Flaherty et al. (1978)		Lindeman et al. (1971) King et al. (1982)	Lindeman et al. (1971) King et al. (1982)
S/P/C		Johnson et al. (1978)		

KEY
SPC Sensory; Procedural; Coping (combined)
PC   Procedural; Coping (combined)
SC   Sensory; Coping (combined)
C   Coping
S/P/C Sensory; Procedural; Coping (separate packages)

The various nursing studies shown in Table 9.2 also utilised different formats for their information giving procedures. The majority involved nurse researchers in verbal interviews, usually of an informal nature. One study used prepared material as well as informal interviews, and one study used only prepared material (tape recordings). The other studies involved ward or operating room nurses in unstructured verbal information giving and/or structured verbal and prepared material. In the unstructured format, the ward staff were prepared by the researchers, often via the head nurse, as to the kind of information to give, and how to give it, using their own words and initiative. In the structured format, the nurses were again prepared in the use of tape-slide material and accompanying booklets, or in the presentation of structured, verbal material. In only one of these studies was the giving of information monitored, it being the express aim of the other studies to evaluate the unsupervised, unmonitored information-giving of nurses. In the structured format, however, the use of the tape-slide equipment and the administration of the booklets did, in effect, monitor the information giving.

Thus, the opportunity for influencing reactions to stressful events such as surgery through interventions which use these cognitive processes has inspired a number of studies, many by nurses, of ways of preparing patients for surgery. A wide range of post-operative outcomes has been identified and shown to be capable of being significantly influenced by pre-operative information giving and instruction. Although different kinds of information have been given to patients, some studies indicate that differential effects can be obtained for them. There is evidence that the various outcome measures are influenced more effectively by the relevant kind of information. The way in which the information is given does not seem to be so important, significant effects being obtained for all the formats used in the studies discussed, even for unstructured, unsupervised information giving. There would seem, therefore, to be a substantial body of evidence demonstrating that patient outcomes, related to a model of stress reduction involving both physiological and psychological factors, can be significantly influenced by nurses giving pre-operative information.

Implementation

The kind of research that has been undertaken in the field of pre-operative information giving, as reviewed above, can be supported by that in related fields, such as that of Wilson-Barnett and Fordham (1982) in the field of patient investigations, coronary care and hysterectomy. But, even though such findings are becoming available to nurses, the questions posed above must still be asked: can nurses put them into practice and, if so, can they achieve the same effect? This is where nursing demonstrates its identity as a profession, and the nurses show themselves to be professional in the care they offer patients. It has been the purpose of this chapter to show in the literature review that there is now a substantial body of knowledge supporting the clinical importance of planned programmes of patient communication. It could be argued that it is professional negligence to be unaware of such research findings and not to implement them when aware.

In one of a series of articles describing the work of the Nursing Research Unit at the University of Edinburgh, a quasi-experimental project was described which was an attempt to monitor the implementation of pre-operative information giving research findings (Davis, 1981). The project involved eight wards in three hospitals and the nursing staff played a most active role in planning the study. The nature and format of the information were decided in conjunction with the ward staff, and the administrative and educational staff organised in-service training sessions to confirm and practise the necessary interpersonal skills. Much of the data used to monitor and evaluate the exercise were collected by the nurses as part of their everyday documentation. Special rating scales for patients' pain perception, perception of sickness, sleep, fitness, feeling cheerful and other outcomes were developed and used by the researcher (Davis, 1984).

A survey of the patients during the study demonstrated that the nurses were implementing findings by giving the patients, who were undergoing biliary and gastric surgery, information in both verbal and booklet formats. The patients expressed their appreciation of the information and a few would have liked even more (Davis, 1984). Significant influences on patients' post-operative progress were demonstrated, echoing the findings discussed in the literature review, and thus showing that ordinary nurses *can* achieve the same sort of benefits as the researchers (Davis, 1984).

However, it must be emphasised that the exercise was only successful because of the cooperation between researchers, managers, educators and practitioners. The researchers made the information available in a comprehensible form; the managers organised and sanctioned the changes in pre-operative nursing care; educators facilitated the preparation of the nurses in the interpersonal skills necessary; and the ward clinical staff helped to translate the research findings into techniques and content for their own practice. That this could occur in three hospitals, involving inner city teaching hospitals and a rural district hospital, confirms the feasibility of such an exercise. However, there may be constraints on successful implementation (see Chapters 4, 5 and 6), and some of the aspects of the management and education of nursing staff preparatory to the introduction or development of interpersonal skills in the clinical setting are discussed at greater length in other chapters (see Chapters 7, 10 and 11). Also, clinical issues feature strongly. The body of knowledge on which professional practice should be based is growing quite quickly. In some areas it is now such that the problems of implementation cause greater concern than those involved in gathering the knowledge. The translation of theory into practice can be achieved, and has been achieved, but not without the coordinated efforts of åll strands of nursing: management, education, practice and research.

The tautology of the oft-quoted phrase 'research-based profession' must be emphasised: a profession, by definition, must be research-based. Similarly with a 'caring profession': a profession not using the latest information cannot really be caring for its clients. If we do not implement research, we are not a profession and we do not care.

Acknowledgement

The literature reviewed in this chapter was collected for a research project which formed part of the Core Programme of the Nursing Research Unit, University of Edinburgh, funded by the Scottish Home and Health Department. The research project has been completed (1984), and a report on it is available from the Nursing Research Unit, entitled 'Pre-operative information giving: an implementation study'.

References

Abdellah, F.G. (1961) 'Criterion Measures in Nursing', *Nursing Research*, *10*, 21-6
Abdellah, F.G. and Levine, E. (1979) *Better Patient Care Through Nursing Research,* Collier Macmillan : London (2nd edn)
Aydelotte, M.K. (1973) 'Quality Assurance Programs in Nursing: Definition and Problems', paper presented at university of Illinois, Chicago
Bloch, D. (1975) 'Evaluation of Nursing Care in Terms of Process and Outcome', *Nursing Research*, *24*, 256-63
Boore, J.R.P. (1978) *Prescription For Recovery*, RCN: London
Carstairs, V. (1970) *Channels of Communication*, SHHD.

Cartwright, A. (1964) *Human Relations and Hospital Care*, Routledge and Kegan Paul: London

Davis, B.D. (1981) 'Pre-operative Information Giving in Relation to Patient Outcome'. (No. 1 in Series 'Communication in Nursing', Nursing Research Unit, Edinburgh) *Nursing Times*, *77*, 599-601

Davis, B.D. (1982) 'Tell Them Like It Is' *Nursing Mirror*, *154*, 26-8

Davis, B.D. (1983) *Perceptions by Nurses, Doctors and Physiotherapists of Pre-Operative Information Giving*, Report to SHHD (NRU, Edinburgh, Core Programme Project)

Davis, B.D. (1984) *Pre-Operative Information Giving: An Implementation Study*, Report to SHHD (NRU Edinburgh, Core Programme Project)

Donabedian, A. (1970) 'Patient Care Evaluation', *Hospitals*, *44*, 131

Dumas, R.G., and Leonard, R.C. (1963) 'Effects of Nursing on the Incidence of Post-operative Vomiting', *Nursing Research*, *12*, 12-15

Felton, G., Huss, K., Payne, E.A., and Sersic, K. (1976) 'Pre-operative Nursing Intervention With the Patient for Surgery: Outcomes of three alternative approaches', *International Journal Nursing Studies*, *13*, 83-96

Flaherty, G.C., and Fitzpatrick, J.J. (1978) 'Relaxation Technique to Increase Comfort Level of Post-operative Patients: A preliminary study', *Nursing Research*, *27*, 352-5

Fortin, F., and Kirouac, S. (1976) 'A Randomised Controlled Trial of Pre-operative Patient Education', *International Journal of Nursing Studies*, *13*, 11-24

Grypdonck, M., Koene, G., Rodenbach, M.Th., Windey, T., and Blanpain, J.E. (1979) 'Integrating Nursing: A holistic approach to the delivery of nursing care', *International Journal of Nursing Studies*, *16*, 215-30

Hagen, E. (1972) 'Appraising the Quality of Nursing Care', *Nursing Research Conference*, *8*, March, 1-8

Hayward, J. (1975) *Information — A Prescription Against Pain*, RCN: London

Hegyvary, S.I. and Chamings, P.A. (1975) '*Hospital Setting and Patient Care Outcomes*, I and II', *Journal of Nursing Administration*, I, 5, 29-32; II, 5, 36-42

Hilger, E. (1974) 'Developing Nursing Outcome Criteria', *Nursing Clinics of North America*, *9*, 323-30

Horsley, J.A., Crane, J., and Bingle, J.D. (1978) 'Research Utilization as an Organizational Process', *Journal of Nursing Administration*, *8*, 4-6

Hunt, J. (1981) 'Indicators for Nursing Practice: The use of research findings', *Journal of Advanced Nursing*, *6*, 189-94

Janis, I.L. (1958) *Psychological Stress*, Wiley: New York

Johnson, J.E. (1973) 'Effects of Accurate Expectations About Sensations on the Sensory and Distress Components of Pain', *Journal of Personality and Social Psychology*, *27*, 261-75

Johnson, J.E., Kirchhoff, N.I., and Endress, M.P. (1975) 'Altering Children's Distress Behaviour During Orthopaedic Cast Removal', *Nursing Research*, *24*, 404-10

Johnson, J.E., and Leventhal, H. (1974) 'Effects of Accurate Expectations and Behavioral Instructions on Reactions During a Noxious Medical Examination', *Journal of Personality and Social Psychology*, *29*, 710-18

Johnson, J.E., Morrissey, J.F. and Leventhal, H. (1973) 'Psychological Preparation for Endoscopic Examination', *Gastrointestinal Endoscopy*, *19*, 180-2

Johnson, J.E., and Rice, V.H. (1974) 'Sensory and Distress Components of Pain', *Nursing Research*, *23*, 203-8

Johnson, J.E., Rice, V.H., Fuller, S.S., and Endress, M.P. (1978) 'Sensory Information, Instruction in a Coping Strategy and Recovery From Surgery', *Research in Nursing and Health*, *1*, 4-17

King, I., and Tarsitano, B. (1982) 'The Effect of Structured and Unstructured Pre-operative Teaching: A replication', *Nursing Research*, *31*, 324-9

Krueger, J.C., Nelson, A.G., and Nolanin, M.O. (1978) *Nursing Research: Develop-ment, Collaboration and Utilization*, Aspen Systems Corporation; Germantown

Krumme, V.S. (1975) 'The Case for Criterion-Referenced Measurement' *Nursing Outlook, 23*, 764-70

Langer, E.J., Janis, I.L., and Wolfer, J.A. (1975) 'Reduction of Psychological Stress in Surgical Patients', *Journal of Experimental Social Psychology, 11*, 155-65

Langer, E.J., and Michaels, S. (1963) *Life Stress and Mental Health*, Glencoe Free Press: London

Lazarus, R.S. (1966) *Psychological Stress and the Coping Process*, McGraw Hill: New York

Lazarus, R.S. (1971) 'The Concepts of Stress and Disease' in L. Levi (ed.), *Society, Stress and Disease : 1. The Psychological Environment and Psychosomatic Disease,* Oxford University Press: London

Lelean, S.R. (1982) 'The Implementation of Research Findings Into Nursing Practice', *International Journal of Nursing Studies, 19*, 223-30

Lindemann, C.A., and Van Aernam, B. (1971) 'Nursing Intervention With the Presurgi-cal Patient: The effects of structured and unstructured pre-operative teaching', *Nurs-ing Research, 20*, 319-32

Luna, H.Q. (1971) 'The Effects of Varied Types of Nursing Approach on Pain Behaviour After Surgery', *ANPHI Papers, 6*, 7-31

McFarlane, J. (1970) *The Proper Study of the Nurse*, RCN: London

Melzack, R, and Wall, P.D. (1965) 'Pain Mechanisms: A new theory', *Science, 150*, 971-9

Melzack, R., and Torgerson, W.S. (1971) 'On the Language of Pain', *Anaesthesiology, 34*, 50-9

Nolan, M.R.G. (1977) 'Effects of Nursing Intervention in the Operating Room as Recalled on the Third Postoperative Day', *Communicating Nursing Research, 9*

Popham, W.J., and Husek, T.R. (1969) 'Implications of Criterion-Referenced Measure-ment', *Journal of Educational Measurement, 6*, 1-9

Raphael, W. (1977) *Patients and Their Hospitals* (3rd edn), King Edward's Hospital Fund for London: London

Royal Commission on the Health Services (1978) HMSO: London

Schmitt, E.F., and Wooldridge, P.J. (1973) 'Psychological Preparation of Surgical Patients', *Nursing Research, 22*, 108-15

Selye, H. (1956) *The Stress of Life*, McGraw Hill: New York

Smith, R.L., and Horn, B.J. (1973) *Development of Criterion Measures of Nursing Care (A proposal)*, School of Public Health: University of Michigan

Speilberger, C.D. (1966) *Anxiety and Behaviour*, Academic Press: New York

Sternbach, R.A. (1966) *Principles of Psychophysiology*, Academic Press: New York

Taylor, J.W. (1974) 'Measuring the Outcomes of Nursing Care', *Nursing Clinics of North America, 9*, 337-48

Towell, D. and Harries, C. (1979) *Innovation in Patient Care*, Croom Helm: London

Voshall, B. (1980) 'The Effects of Pre-operative Teaching on Post-operative Pain', *Topics in Clinical Nursing, 2*, 39-43

Weddell, A.G.M. (1962) '"Activity Pattern Hypothesis" for Sensation of Pain' in R.G. Grenell (ed.), *Progress in Neurobiology, Vol. 5: Neuralphysiopathology*, Hoeber: New York

Wilson-Barnett, J. (1978) *Stress in Hospital*, Churchill Livingstone: Edinburgh

Wilson-Barnett, J., and Fordham, M. (1982) *Recovery from Illness*, Wiley: London

Zimmer, M.J. (1974) 'Guidelines for Development of Outcome Criteria', *Nursing Clinics of North America, 9*, 317-21

PART IV:

INTERPERSONAL SKILLS IN SPECIFIC NURSING CONTEXTS

EDITORIAL INTRODUCTION

Whether or not nurses *do* lack key interpersonal skills partly depends on the type of interaction that is expected or possible. Nursing care is complex and there is a diversity of models of nursing used to dictate the nature and practice of care. These range from those that emphasise high technology to those that emphasise the humanistic nature of nursing. Patients, too, have different needs with regard to nursing care, depending on their state of health and the nature of their disabilities.

In *Chapter 10*, *Pat Ashworth* draws attention to the case of interpersonal skill needs in intensive care units. Here, patients may have restricted ability to express themselves, high physical dependence and restrictions, low self-esteem and disorientation. Staff are working in a high pressure area that is often emotionally charged: there may be strained relationships with colleagues, special requirements to pass information to each other and to communicate with relatives. Ashworth describes the physical and psychosocial barriers that nurses, patients and relatives might have, that could inhibit effective communication. She suggests that nurses may need to decide, consciously, to use different channels of communication with their patients, in order to stimulate them. This places somewhat unusual demands on the nurses, who have to try to be especially creative in their use of interpersonal skill in this high technology environment. Ashworth advocates training along experiential lines as a means of preparing and equipping nurses to use appropriate interpersonal skills in intensive care settings.

Mastectomy nursing offers a stark contrast to work in intensive care. *Ann Tait*, in *Chapter 11*, reminds us that the very mention of cancer in our society is taboo, and this, coupled with challenges to body image and self-esteem causes a great deal of trauma to mastectomy patients, nurses and relatives. The skills that nurses need to develop are those that enable them to 'get close' to their patients so that they are able to detect psychosocial effects of the disease. Tait describes specialist nurse projects that have successfully trained nurses in these assessment skills, using pragmatic, directive methods with systematic feedback. Skilled assessment has led to greater social recovery of patients with little effect on physical disability. Similar successes have been achieved by ward and community nurses. A by-product of gaining competence in the ability to assess patients' coping capacity and to identify problems, has been an increase in the extent of personal support that the nurses themselves need. In the project that Tait was involved with this was freely available, but she notes that if it were not, the stress that nurses would then be likely to experience would detract from the possibilities for personal growth that derive from working with this group of patients.

10 INTERPERSONAL SKILL ISSUES ARISING FROM INTENSIVE CARE NURSING CONTEXTS

Pat Ashworth

Introduction

Competence in nursing skills is usually highly valued and much sought after by intensive care nurses, and rightly so since it may have considerable influence on both the short-term and long-term wellbeing or even survival of their patients. Interpersonal skills are amongst the most crucial since, unless the nurses can use these, neither they and their patients, nor patients' visitors and other staff, can fully use their resources to benefit the patients. Yet until recently these skills were rarely included in either basic or post-basic education in nursing in the UK. Even if the ability to communicate with patients was valued by some nurses it was usually assumed that this was either innate, or could be 'caught' by working with other experienced nurses but not taught, as are other skills, with a basis of knowledge.

Objectives concerned with communication with patients, relatives and staff were included in the Outline Curriculum for the Joint Board of Clinical Nursing Studies Intensive Care Nursing Course from the time it was designed around 1972, as they later were in other courses. Yet in 1978, two members of the Joint Board staff initiated a Communication Studies Group because of evidence received by the Board that 'the communication objective within the curricula, which is placed second only in importance to the clinical skills in the majority of courses, was not being taught in any specific or structured way in most of the courses. Moreover the majority of the teaching staff involved with the JBCNS courses had little idea how this subject could be incorporated into their teaching programmes.' The teaching staff had received little preparation for teaching the subject, and had little knowledge of appropriate teaching methods (Bridge and Speight, 1981).

In recent years there have been several studies of nurse-patient communication in various clinical areas in the UK, for example studies relating to medical (Faulkner, 1984), surgical (Macleod Clark, 1983), geriatric (Wells, 1980) and cancer (Bond, 1983) patients. These are in many ways relevant to the consideration of interpersonal nursing skills in intensive care units, since any of such patients are to be found in intensive care units. Furthermore, intensive care nurses have usually had the same kind of educational preparation (or lack of it) in the use of interpersonal skills as have other nurses. They are likely to have been socialised in similar ways into similar communication patterns. These studies, and others reviewed by their respective authors, seem to provide a composite picture of nurse-patient communication patterns characterised by short interactions, focused largely on physical aspects of care and treatment and providing little relevant, consistent and specific information or effective emotional support in distress. Patients' questions, whether direct or oblique, seemed to be discouraged rather than encouraged, and often met with responses which appeared unhelpful. Macleod Clark (1983, p.32) perceptively states that

> The fact that patients appear to consciously adopt a passive role, perceiving the nurses as 'busy' and 'not to be worried' is important. If this is the case, the responsibility for taking the initiative in encouraging patients to discuss problems and anxieties falls even more to the nurses.

If these are findings with patients who can talk and are in the relatively 'normal' surroundings of hospital wards, what about nurse-patient communication in intensive care units?

Perhaps some of the most important issues to be considered in relation to communication in intensive care units are:

How does interpersonal interaction in an intensive care unit differ from that in other areas?
What are the main purposes of communication there?
What are the actual and potential barriers to communication?
What skills are needed to overcome these barriers?
How can these skills best be developed and their use in practice encouraged?

Communication in Intensive Care Units

Whenever one person is in contact with another, information is exchanged unless total unconsciousness makes this impossible. The information may be transmitted verbally or non-verbally by use of signals conveyed, for example, by facial expression, eye contact, touch, body movements and posture, and other non-verbal aspects of speech, vocal tone, proximity and appearance (Argyle, 1975). When verbal and non-verbal messages are not congruent it tends to be the non-verbal message that is received. Blondis and Jackson (1982) suggest that use of time also conveys messages; time spent with a patient when no procedure is performed may communicate interest and caring. Non-verbal signals not only convey messages but may also be used deliberately or unconsciously to reinforce or amplify verbal messages, to convey emotions and to regulate interaction. For example, most people tend to look at other people while listening, may look away while speaking, but then look at them again when they are about to stop speaking (Argyle, 1975). Most people actively seek information about others in order to know what they can expect of them (Goffman, 1959), have an image of how they appear to others, and may make considerable effort to present a particular image. Often there is a shared understanding of the situation which reduces the amount of information which must be conveyed. Hall (1983) shows how, with an increase in existing shared understanding (high context communication), the amount of information which must be transmitted decreases, and vice versa (Figure 10.1). Usually people are simultaneously both sending and receiving messages and feedback; the reception of information about how others are responding to one's communication is very important. Lack of feedback is often so disconcerting that it may lead to disruption, diminution or even cessation of verbal communication. Other factors such as role relationships and the physical and social environment also affect interpersonal interaction.

It is evident that full and effective use of all communication channels requires the physical, emotional and intellectual capacity to send signals which convey their intended meaning and to receive them, and also some common understanding with those with whom it is sought to communicate. But this is precisely what most patients in intensive care units often do not have. All are restricted in their ability to express themselves by body movement and personal appearance. They are usually unfamiliar with being in a situation where they are physically dependent on other people; where bodily functions usually performed independently in private require assistance and/or permission, and are matters for relatively public discussion; and where they may not understand the physical objects, activities and sounds (including much of the verbal interchange) around them. They need information about their own condition, and the environment and expectations; yet in order

Figure 10.1

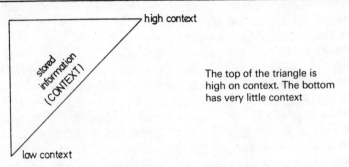

The top of the triangle is high on context. The bottom has very little context

Pair this triangle with another in a balanced relationship. In this second triangle there is very little information at the top and more at the bottom.

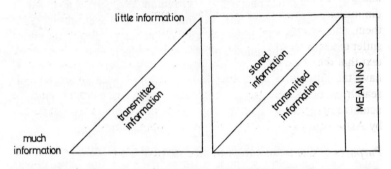

Source: *The Dance of Life* by Edward T. Hall Copyright 1983 by Edward T. Hall, Reprinted by permission of Brandt & Brandt Literary Agents, Inc.

to conform to traditional expectations of the 'good patient' (seen as passive and undemanding), and because they do not feel confident of knowing the right words to use, they are often unwilling or unable to pressure staff to provide it. Staff do not always provide the necessary longer-term/orienting information spontaneously (Ashworth, 1980); and since nurses in other clinical areas in the UK gave inappropriate or discouraging responses to about half of all patients' questions (Macleod Clark, 1984) or inaccurate or very limited information (Faulkner, 1984) it is likely that this may occur in intensive care units also. The patients' self-esteem may be diminished by illness and dependency, thus making them unwilling or unable to persist in their efforts to gain the information they need.

Many intensive care unit patients have additional problems in that they cannot speak, because of endotracheal tubes; are limited in their reception of communication by dressings, equipment, lack of visual aids, or other impediments to sensory function (hearing, sight), and in interpretation of messages received owing to disturbed mental function. They may be unable to convey any non-verbal messages deliberately owing to paralysis of pathological, traumatic or pharmacological origin, and thus can provide no feedback to others attempting to communicate with them. They may suffer disorientation, hallucination and other symptoms of disorientation and consequently have a totally different frame of reference from those who are in contact with them.

Staff, too, are affected by the intensive care unit situation, which may affect their use of interpersonal skills. They are often working under pressure in anxiety-provoking situations, where there may be role relationship problems with doctors and other staff (Edelstein, 1966) and where their own self-esteem and self-confidence may at times be diminished by inadequate educational preparation for the demands on them, and feelings of guilt and inadequacy particularly when patients suffer excessively or die (Cassem and Hackett, 1975). It is in this context that they face the problems of communicating with patients who have the difficulties described above. (Further information and research on communication, the intensive care environment, and the actual or potential effects of both can be found in reviews such as those by Ashworth, 1980; 1984a; 1984b; and other authors.)

Purposes of Communication in an Intensive Care Unit

Ceccio and Ceccio (1982) suggest that four basic communication objectives are: to inquire, to inform, to persuade, to entertain. However, it seems that these can be expanded and made more explicit in relation to communication in intensive care units. As a result of a literature review and interviews with patients and staff (Ashworth, 1980), four main aims for nurse-patient communication were defined:

(1) To establish a relationship in which patients perceive nurses as friendly, helpful, competent and reliable, and as recognising the patients' worth and individuality.

(2) To try to determine the patients' needs as perceived by them, themselves, and when necessary to help them recognise their other needs, as perceived by the nurse.

(3) To provide factual information by which the patients can structure their expectations.

(4) To assist the patients to use their own resources and those offered to them (e.g. information) to meet their own needs.

Purposes and aims of communication between staff in the intensive care unit include: transmission and exchange of information necessary to maintain or increase the patients' structural and physiological, personal and social integrity, and maintain continuity of care; organisational communication necessary for the continuous supply of human and other resources, warning of hazards etc.; and interpersonal interaction necessary for the maintenance of working relationships and mutual support in stressful situations. While the first two of these are usually recognised and mechanisms are provided to achieve them, the third is sometimes not considered adequately and is left to chance.

Communication with patients' visitors tends to be controlled by staff, and therefore also needs consideration if it is to be adequate. Three of the main aims of communication between staff and visitors are: to enable the visitor to provide the greatest possible help and support to their family member/friend; to prevent the visitor suffering unduly from the situation; and to enable the visitor to cooperate with staff, to the benefit of all concerned.

These aims and purposes are not always easy to achieve, but identification of them and of the actual or potential barriers to communication are the first necessary steps towards doing so. The interpersonal skills necessary to achieve the purposes can then be assessed and, if necessary, learned.

Barriers to Accurate and Helpful Communication

Communication between Nurses and Patients

Actual or potential barriers to nurse-patient communication can be summarised in relation to four main areas (see Figure 10.2): the patients as senders and receivers of messages, and the nurses as senders and receivers of messages. This is complicated by the fact that in each interaction each patient and nurse is involved both as the person he or she perceives himself or herself to be, and as the person perceived by others, and the perceptions may be different. The barriers to interaction may be physical or psychosocial. Barriers originating in patients as senders and receivers of messages may include:

physical factors — such as dysphasia or aphonia, limited movement, strength and control impeding writing, gestures and reaching out to touch;

Figure 10.2: Nurse-Patient Communication

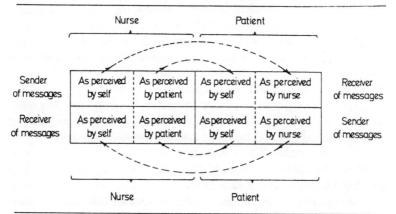

		Nurse		Patient		
Sender of messages	As perceived by self	As perceived by patient	As perceived by self	As perceived by nurse	Receiver of messages
Receiver of messages	As perceived by self	As perceived by patient	As perceived by self	As perceived by nurse	Sender of messages
		Nurse		Patient		

— lack of, or distorted, facial expression and possibly eye contact, due to paralysis, injury or other pathology, or equipment e.g. maxillary fixation splints or endotracheal tube;

— impairment of sensory reception (due to defects in vision, hearing etc.), preventing full reception and understanding, and affecting messages sent by preventing feedback on the nurses' response to previous signals from the patient;

— cerebral function impairment due to trauma, hypoxia or other such causes.

psychosocial factors — such as anxiety and uncertainty, perception of total dependence, and lack of information about the environment and the people in it;

— role relationship expectations which do not match those of the nurses e.g. expectation that nurses will always be gentle and comforting and patients allowed to rest, when in reality it may be necessary for nurses to interrupt rest and perform or help the patient to perform procedures which may be uncomfortable, such as coughing and aspiration of secretions after thoracic surgery;

— impaired intellectual function due to drugs, sensory deprivation, excessive stressful factors or other such causes, which may prevent accurate interpretation of messages from others and appropriate responses;

— impaired self-concept, depression and a sense of helplessness, hopelessness and lack of progress; or frustration and aggression against their dependency and others' perceived lack of concern or respect for their values, privacy and dignity.

Barriers originating with nurses may include:

physical barriers — such as wearing a mask which makes speech less distinct and hides facial expression;

— physical characteristics, mannerisms or behaviours which may be anxiety-provoking or intimidating; for example a large, strong, serious-looking nurse may be intimidating or provide security and comfort, depending on other verbal and/or non-verbal behaviour. The patients' perception of height and other characteristics may be distorted by their position; and they may perceive as threatening a set facial expression which is in reality due to the nurse's preoccupation or anxiety. A smile and personal comment may counteract this.

psychosocial factors — such as preoccupation with tasks and other work of varying intensity and urgency;

— sense of frustration, worry, inadequacy, embarrassment or other negative feelings when communication is difficult;

— the difficulty of talking to an unresponsive person or one who does not provide rewarding responses, e.g. appreciation and social interaction, which motivate further communication;

— difficulty in overcoming patients' impaired sensory function;

— difficulty in talking to someone about whom little or nothing is known other than current medical condition, observable characteristics and behaviour;

— beliefs and values that 'the work' (task) is more important than responding to the patients' emotional and personal needs, or that interaction with ill patients should be minimised so that they are 'left to rest' (the presumption being that they will rest if left alone: this is not always an accurate assumption);

— concern that attempting to communicate may cause an artificially-ventilated patient who is 'settled' to breathe out of synchrony with the machine, which may be harmful to them: (this is a less common problem now that machines which accommodate the patient's own breathing efforts are more often in use);

— the nurses' own feelings of tiredness, anxiety, need for protection from further emotional demands;

— deficiency in educational preparation and continuing support to provide security in dealing with the emotional demands and communication requirements of patients, their visitors, other staff and themselves.

In addition to all these barriers there is the complication that the people with whom the nurses interact (defined by them according to their knowledge and observations of their condition and communication ability, behaviour, personality and other characteristics) may not be the same as the people the patients perceive themselves to be (with their current sensations and experience interpreted in the light of past experiences, knowledge, self-image and ways of coping and responding to stressors). For example nurses may interact with patients whom they perceive to be dependent, slow to comprehend and limited in understanding, with possible cerebral damage; whereas the patients may have recovered sufficiently to understand and think relatively clearly but take time to work out how to express themselves and their difficulty in doing things, because of their tracheostomy. (In one situation like this the patient later said to a nurse researcher, 'The nurses roar at you. They don't give you time.') Sometimes when nurses care for unresponsive patients over time with little knowledge of them as people they endow them with personalities which prove to be very different from their own, which become evident as they recover.

Or the patients may perceive 'their' nurse (i.e. a succession of people who may in their mind be confused) as people who constantly do strange and/or uncomfortable things to them, e.g. tracheal suction, injections and making them cough, which may be painful with an endotracheal tube, and whose intentions may or may not be friendly. As one patient put it (after 5 weeks of curarisation and artificial ventilation, and subsequent recovery):

> Towards the end they seemed to take a particular interest in getting me on my feet, and goading me into it. I couldn't understand it at the time. I thought they were a little like children, like cats, playing with mice. I thought perhaps they'd taken a dislike to me . . .. I couldn't make up my mind whether they were helping me or they were playing with me . . . (Ashworth, 1976)

If patients have become disorientated they may be 'living in another world', where the people around may not be perceived as hospital staff and visitors and the environment seems to be something very different from a hospital unit. Patients who remember little or nothing else about the intensive care unit may report such experiences if asked whether they suffered strange dreams or nightmares while ill (Ashworth, 1976), and often these experiences can be related to misinterpreted events and situations in the intensive care unit. Many experienced intensive care nurses have found that patients recognise the individual nurses' voices after discharge from the unit, even though they do not recognise the nurses' appearance, and this aspect of communication obviously makes an impact even on apparently unconscious patients.

Communication Between Staff

Communication between staff may be impeded by the pressure of work and difficulty in finding time to communicate adequately without interruptions and a sense of haste. Much information must be exchanged concisely, precisely and accurately, but this requires skills which must be learned, particularly as written communication must be used to complement or replace verbal interaction. Communication may also be complicated by interpersonal relationships, which may be a source of great stress or great satisfaction in intensive care units (Claus and Bailey, 1980). Those who manage to convey to others a sense of respect and warmth, despite the pressured circumstances at times, can do much to improve staff-staff relationships. But at times when things are not going well and patients die, as inevitably some do, staff may suffer from feelings of failure, guilt and diminished self-esteem, and this may lead to a tendency to 'blaming' and friction unless the feelings can be acknowledged.

There is also potential friction between very experienced intensive care nurses who know a great deal about medical as well as nursing aspects of the work, and doctors who may be relatively inexperienced in intensive care yet retain the prescribing role. The doctors may feel that they know, or should know, all about assessing and treating the patient and take the lead and give orders. The experienced nurses may recognise that they are in a three-sided 'bind'. If they suggest what should be done, the doctors may reject both their suggestions and themselves as colleagues; if they do not say anything the patients may suffer; in addition, they may be criticised later by more senior medical staff for not having done something about the situation. Nurses, too, sometimes fail to accept and acknowledge the expertise of other health workers. In the midst of all the other complications there is great potential for misinterpretation of non-verbal signals with unfortunate consequences. For example, the doctor's frown and abruptness as she/he arrives on the unit may provoke a similar response from the unit staff, who may perceive her/him as cross and irritable, rather than tired and worried, which may be the actual cause of her/his behaviour. Or the same kind of thing may happen in reverse when the nurses are tired and overstretched.

Communication Between Staff and Visitors

Communication and relationships between staff and their patients' families or other visitors may be mutually supportive, or stressful to staff and unsatisfactory to the visitors (Dunkel and Eisendrath, 1983).

Some of the major barriers to communication between staff and visitors appear to be:
— the different knowledge, understanding, frames of reference and vocabularies of staff and visitors. What is familiar and simple to staff may be strange, unintelligible, or just plain terrifying to visitors;
— the real or apparent busyness and attitude of staff which may make visitors hesitant to approach them for information or help;
— visitors' anxiety which may limit their ability to understand quickly what is said;
— visitors' sensory deficits — some visitors are elderly and may not hear or see well;
— lack of recognition by the staff that visitors have a positive contribution to make to patient welfare and that, for this reason, as well as other humanitarian ones, they merit thoughtful attention from staff.

Skills Necessary for Effective Interpersonal Interaction in Intensive Care Units

The first essential general skills for effective interpersonal interaction in intensive care units are *assessment skills*. These require application of knowledge of basic channels and methods of communication to each particular situation to assess which are still available to the patient, which are impaired but could easily be improved, which are inevitably not available at least in the near future, and what could be done to improve impaired function and/or use alternative channels. This includes considering such questions as:
— Can the patients speak or write? Can they hear? Can they understand the nurses' language (national language and the type of words used)? Do they use a hearing aid?
— Can they open their eyes? If they are open (by their own volition or with assistance) can they see? Do they usually use spectacles or contact lenses? Can they read?
— Can they move to make signals or reach out to touch? Or are they physically unable to do so, or afraid to move because of attached equipment, pain, fear, or belief that it may not be permissible?
— If unable to talk do they have preferred ways of attracting attention or communicating, and if so what do these signs mean? Blondis and Jackson (1982) describe in detail an example of how the nursing process was used to improve a young paralysed man's communication

with other staff who found his constant 'clicking' with his tongue to attract attention infuriating and stressful, and yet it later transpired that he had been taught by other nurses to call them in this way.

Børsig and Steinacker (1982) provide a good diagrammatic analysis for the assessment of various channels of communication. Assessment must include not only the patient's ability to receive and transmit messages, but also the human and physical environment and situation, which may affect not only the communication needed, but also the way in which the patient interacts.

The specific skills necessary to assess adequately include observation skills, critical thinking and problem-solving. It is not enough to observe that the patient cannot do something or is in an undesirable emotional state (e.g. acute anxiety or aggression). It is necessary to think beyond those observations to the reasons behind them; that is, to identify the basic problem, and whether it is potentially soluble. Verbal skills such as open-ended questions ('How are you feeling?') rather than closed, yes-no questions, or leading questions ('You're feeling better aren't you?') can be useful in assessment; and the skills of clarifying, and reflecting back (Long and Prophit, 1981) are often necessary to check the accuracy of observations, though the nurse may have to manage with non-verbal responses from those patients who cannot talk.

Much of what has been said is just as applicable to communication with other staff and visitors as it is with patients. One essential factor in good interpersonal interaction is self-awareness, but not acute self-consciousness which inhibits communication. This means learning to be sensitive to one's own effect on the interaction, and the possible reasons for this. These reasons may include intrapersonal factors such as prejudices, fears or stress. For example Bond (1982) suggests that behavioural reactions to stress may include saying provocative things, arguing, or non-verbal aggression. Or one may provoke aggression or even assault by failing to respect someone's personal space, e.g. by doing something to a patient and invading their privacy without adequate explanation or permission (Maagdenberg, 1983). Dominating communication may provoke resistance even in otherwise docile and compliant people, whether the recipient is a staff member, patient or visitor. Similarly, defensive communication may provoke defensive listening, and a cycle of increasingly distorted perceptions (Gibb, 1982).

Having identified potential barriers and problems in communication, the content and messages that need to be conveyed and possible ways of overcoming barriers, the next general skills needed are those of *setting the objectives* to be achieved by communication and *planning* ways of achieving them. Skills such as clarifying and reflecting back are often still important at the intervention stage. But alongside these there are other essential skills such as nurturing ('mothering' and encouraging the person), and supporting (showing unconditional regard for the person, 'being there' and helping the person through bad patches) which Tschudin (1982) describes in counselling. These are equally essential when caring for intensive care patients who may endure prolonged or frequent 'bad patches'. They need nurses who will sustain them emotionally as well as physically, assisting them to regain their own confidence and independence as this becomes possible. It is important to listen carefully since often there are several messages in what is said. For example, there may be knowledge (cognitive), emotional (affective) and experiential content (Long and Prophit, 1981), and it may help the person more if one responds to one of these rather than another, or responds to each in turn. For example, if a patient with a tracheostomy gets agitated and writes 'Why do you keep sticking those tubes down my throat? It makes my chest hurt and I can't breathe. It scares me stiff,' he/she needs more than an explanation of why tracheal suction is necessary. He/she also needs an acknowledgement of his/her fear and distress, an assurance that the nurse will keep him/her safe, and teaching on how best to help him/herself and reduce the discomfort.

For many intensive care patients the nurses' skills in non-verbal communication are very important. Deliberate touch such as holding the patient's hand, or a hand on his/her shoulder, can be very important as a means of complementing or even replacing speech at times. Because of their dependence, intensive care patients are often very sensitive to non-verbal communication, such as tone of voice, touch or facial expression. This means that nurses need to be very aware of what they may be conveying, and use these channels deliberately, particularly if some channels are limited. For example, if a patient cannot see, additional verbal description of the situation, tone of voice and touch must often be used more, and it may be useful to guide the patient's hand to feel some equipment so that he/she understands what is attached to him/her and why.

Planning the content of information needed by patients and the speed at which they can cope with it are also necessary skills. This requires knowledge of essential requirements, such as orienting information about the people and environment that surround them; why they are in the unit and what is being done to help them; possibly, how long they may be in the unit if that is known; and when their visitors may be arriving and who has enquired. Some purely social conversation can be helpful, provided that it concerns things which interest the patients and involve them as people. A number of ex-patients, including a Professor of Anaesthetics, have said that they sometimes enjoyed hearing staff socially communicate with each other, so long as the patient is included by verbal comment or non-verbally in the interaction and not 'talked over' and ignored. Methods of conveying the information and other content may include verbal and non-verbal methods as appropriate, and may sometimes include pictures, diagrams or taped music or other sounds. These may help if patients need to be reoriented to their own identity and past life; for example, a young fireman recovering after a head injury was helped by his colleagues who came and played to him tapes of sounds heard in the fire station, and talked about their work together.

It is also useful to give some consideration to communication between staff, and the skills necessary to achieve good and effective interpersonal working relationships. Communication of messages about patient care or organisation matters must usually be clear, concise and explicit if it is to be effective. But speaking or writing messages of this kind are skills which often require conscious thought and practice initially, and intermittent review. The possible emotional impact of a message is important as well as the informative, prescriptive or descriptive content. A message which is clear, concise and explicit when conveyed verbally with a smile and other warm, respectful non-verbal signals may appear abrupt or impersonal, or even rude, if conveyed in writing in some contexts, and may not produce the desired response. Or it may produce an undesired response. The nature of interpersonal communication generally between staff is important — is it supportive and helpful, and does it promote development? Do people have and use the interpersonal skills, verbal and non-verbal, to provide each other with positive 'strokes' (Berne, 1976)? Edwards & Brilhart (1981) suggest that the self-concepts of the participants are major components of the communication, and this certainly seems to be so in practice. So often, particularly in stressful situations, staff make explicit the negative messages about performance to each other but not the positive ones. This may happen when a person already feels inadequate in a difficult situation and may result in an even more negative self-concept, which may cause withdrawal or defensiveness, which in turn lead to more negative responses.

How can Interpersonal Skills be Learned or Improved?

The first step is to become conscious of the ways in which messages are conveyed from one person to another. Although most people are aware that non-verbal communication occurs, many nurses have never analysed in how many ways this can occur. A group 'brainstorming' session is one way of doing this analysis, and may be more helpful than just reading a list in a book. A useful next step may be to listen and observe what actually happens in interpersonal interaction in an intensive care unit. This may be difficult to do at first while actually involved in the situation, particularly in emergency. But it is sometimes possible when one is less busy to stop and think 'What can I hear? What does the tone of voice, speed of speech, etc. tell me? What do the facial expressions, body positions and gestures of the speakers and listeners convey? How would this affect me if I were one of the participants in the interaction? How might a patient react to this interaction?', and other such questions. Another way of doing this sort of analysis is to use videotapes which can be viewed by a group. The group leader may then show a section of tape and ask the group to answer the same sort of questions as those just suggested. Videotapes of this kind are available commercially, but none so far shows intensive care situations. The purpose is not to say what someone did wrong and allocate blame, but to identify what is happening and the possible effects, and consider alternatives. Or one of the group may describe an incident which can then be analysed, including the participants' feelings, the possible effects, and alternative ways of handling the situation.

Role-play can be useful and offers an opportunity for the participants not only to analyse what happened, but also to give each other feedback on how they felt. It may be more difficult to role play intubated patients with limb paralysis who cannot talk and are trying to convey that they have a pain in a specific place, but it can be done, and may evoke the kind of frustration in both participants which occurs in real situations. In role-play it is possible to discuss this, and try out alternative ways of coping with the situation to see which seems most useful to both 'patient' and nurse. The opportunity to try out different interventions in a 'safe' situation without risk to a patient may make nurses more confident in trying out new or different skills in real situations. Anne Tomlinson (Chapter 12) discusses various forms of experiential learning and some of the techniques that can usefully be employed.

Experiential learning may take place in a classroom with, for example, nurse-'patients', with their eyes covered, being moved around without warning, or 'talked over' and ignored. Or exercises may be planned to help participants to realise that direct eye contact, close physical proximity and touch may be too overwhelming in some circumstances and for some cultures, while for others they may be helpful. Experiential learning may also take place in an actual intensive care unit. Many intensive care nurses have said how much they learned from being a patient or visiting a friend or relative in such a unit. Obviously this is not experience one would plan to give to nurses. But one can plan to help them (or oneself) to learn by listening to those who have had such experience, either in class or more informally from staff and patients in the unit; or by reading books recording such experiences. Talking to patients after transfer from an intensive care unit can be very informative, and they are sometimes able to say what they found most helpful or most unhelpful. But many of the patients who spend longest in a unit and perhaps are artificially ventilated say afterwards that they cannot remember it. Yet they may have been disoriented and 'living in a nightmare' during the experience, and may talk about this if encouraged to do so. It is perhaps particularly important for them that intensive care nurses take every opportunity during their care to observe their response to the situation in the unit, and to offer them the opportunity to talk or use the other means of self-expression to describe their perception of the experience. With greater understanding of their patients' perceptions, nurses can plan to use their interpersonal skills more effectively to the patients' advantage and learn from the response. What is learned from one patient may be used to help others, though individual assessment is always necessary. No two people are exactly alike.

Learning interpersonal skills does not mean that those who have learned will always practise them perfectly in the future, any more than learning to drive a car means constantly perfect driving. Habits develop in anything one does constantly. But repeated review and constructively critical evaluation, or self-evaluation, of interpersonal skills can develop 'good habits' and more personal and mutually rewarding communication, and inhibit 'bad habits'. One can learn what sorts of circumstances are likely to make one communicate ineffectively, whether due to prejudice, anxiety or other personal feelings, or particular circumstances. If these are acknowledged then it is possible to plan more constructive ways of dealing with the situation and achieve better communication.

Some people come into nursing with better-developed social skills than others. But all need to consider and learn to use interpersonal skills deliberately in professional practice, with awareness of possible impediments and consequences. Good interpersonal skills can best be learned, used and developed in a social environment where each person respects and is respected by others, and each contributes to the 'building up' of others. Such an environment does not usually occur by accident in the demanding and sometimes stressful situation of an intensive care unit. It requires effort, and since nurses are the people most constantly present with patients, visitors and other staff, they probably have most influence as to whether it is achieved or not.

Despite the pressure of many other things to learn, it is worth spending time and effort to teach and learn good interpersonal skills. Experience in the demanding and sometimes stressful and dramatic circumstances in an intensive care unit can impair a person and their effective functioning, whether patient (Kiely, 1973), visitor or staff (Cassem and Hackett, 1975). So for utilitarian as well as humanitarian reasons the human aspects of intensive care cannot be ignored without cost. Many, probably most, staff *do* care about people. Good interpersonal skills can be used to convey this care, and develop supportive relationships which can help to transform potentially very negative experiences into ones of growth and development.

References

Argyle, (1975) *Bodily Communication*, Methuen; London

Ashworth, P. (1976) 'An Investigation into Problems of Communication Between Nurses and Patients in Intensive Therapy/Care Units', unpublished MSc thesis University of Manchester

Ashworth, P. (1980) *Care to Communicate: An investigation into problems of communication between patients and nurses in intensive therapy units*. RCN: London

Ashworth, P. (1984a) 'Communicating in an intensive care unit' in: A. Faulkner (ed.), *Recent Advances in Nursing*; 7, *Communication*, Churchill Livingstone : Edinburgh

Ashworth, P. (1984b) 'Staff-patient Communication in Coronary Care Units', *Journal of Advanced Nursing*, *9*, 35-42

Berne, E. (1976) *Games People Play*, Penguin: Harmondsworth

Blondis, M.N. and Jackson, B.E. (1982) *Non-verbal Communication with Patients*, Wiley: New York (2nd edn)

Bond, M. (1982) 'Self-awareness', *Nursing Mirror*, 29 September, 26-9

Bond, S. (1983) 'Nurses' Communication with Cancer Patients' in J. Wilson-Barnett (ed.), *Nursing Research: Ten Studies in Patient Care*, Wiley: London

Børsig, A. and Steinacker, I. (1982) 'Communication with the Patient in the Intensive Care Unit', *Nursing Times Supplement*, 24 March. 1-11

Bridge, W. and Speight, I. (1981) 'Teaching the Skills of Nursing Communication', *Nursing Times*, Occasional Paper, 18 November, 125-7

Cassem, N.H. and Hackett, T.P. (1975) 'Stress on the Nurse and Therapist in the Intensive Care Unit and Coronary Care Unit', *Heart & Lung*, *4*, 252-9

Ceccio, J.F. and Ceccio, C.M. (1982) *Effective Communication in Nursing: Theory and Practice*, Wiley: New York

Claus, K. and Bailey, J.T. (1980) *Living with Stress and Promoting Well-Being*, Mosby: S. Louis

Dunkel, J. and Eisendrath, S. (1983) 'Families in the Intensive Care Unit: their effect on staff', *Heart and Lung, 12,* 258-61

Edelstein, R. (1966) 'Automation — its Effect on the Nurse', *American Journal of Nursing*, *66,* 2194-8

Edwards, B.J. and Brilhart, J.K. (1981) *Communication in Nursing Practice*, Mosby: St Louis

Faulkner, A. (ed.) (1984) *Recent Advances in Nursing, 7, Communication*, Churchill Livingstone: Edinburgh

Gibb, J.R. (1982) 'Defensive Communication', *Journal of Nursing Administration*, *82,* 14-17

Goffman, E. (1959) *The Presentation of Self in Everyday Life*, Penguin Books: Harmondsworth (1971)

Hall, E.T. (1983) *The Dance of Life: The Other Dimension of Time*, Anchor Press/Doubleday: New York

Kiely, W.F. (1973) 'Critical Care Psychiatric Syndromes', *Heart and Lung*, *2,* 54-7

Long, L. and Prophit, P. (1981) *Understanding/Responding: A Communication Manual for Nurses*, Wadsworth Health Sciences Division: California

Maagdenberg, A.M. (1983) 'The 'Violent' Patient', *American Journal of Nursing*, March, 402-3

Macleod Clark, J. (1983) 'Nurse-Patient Communication: An analysis of conversations from surgical wards' in J. Wilson-Barnett (ed.), *Nursing Research: Ten Studies in Patient Care*, Wiley: London

Macleod Clark, J. (1984) 'Verbal Communication in Nursing' A. Faulkner (ed.) *Recent Advances in Nursing, 7, Communication*, Churchill Livingstone : Edinburgh

Tschudin, V. (1982) *Counselling Skills for Nurses*, Bailliere Tindall: London

Wells, T.J. (1980) *Problems in Geriatric Nursing Care*, Churchill Livingstone: Edinburgh

11 INTERPERSONAL SKILL ISSUES ARISING FROM MASTECTOMY NURSING CONTEXTS

Ann Tait

Introduction

On commonsense grounds alone, good interpersonal skills would seem to be important in the nursing care of patients with breast cancer. If we are to look at the particular issues raised by research in this field, our understanding as to why they arise may be helped by looking at the broader context in which commonsense and research based views are reached, for this is a context that we all help to construct. Where breast cancer is concerned, the issues raised are peculiarly emotive, have unique connotations and can pose distinctive kinds of threat. There are several reasons for this.

The Context of Breast Cancer

The Facts

In the United Kingdom any woman has a 1 in 14 chance of developing breast cancer; it is the leading cause of death for women between 35 and 54 years of age. Over 12,000 women die of this disease each year and the annual incidence has been increasing at the rate of 1 per cent. Also mortality rates have not changed significantly for 30 years (Baum, 1981). The feeling of threat to life, therefore, has a rational basis. However, it could be argued that only 4 per cent of women as a whole die from breast cancer in this country, whereas 22 per cent die from coronary disease. So why the distinctive concern?

Cancer

Because the aetiology of cancer is unknown and yet treatments proliferate, the characteristics of cancer are surrounded by an aura of mystification — even the word cancer is symbolic of death itself and is the standardised nightmare of our time (Sontag, 1979). Cancer also serves as an emotionally charged metaphor for the inexplicable (Comaroff and Maguire, 1981). As well as the ever present threat to life

165

there can be stigma, guilt and shame, with puzzlement at what often appears to be an unheralded and undeserved catastrophe. Cancer is unique among illnesses in the deep rooted fear it evokes (Weisman, 1979), and the patient is under a special and unusually severe form of stress (Mastrovito, 1972).

These fears and stresses are not confined to patients. In the 1960s, nurses were found to be unduly pessimistic about the curability of cancer (Davison, 1965). In the 1980s the picture has hardly improved. Only a minority of trained nurses could predict accurate survival rates for differing stages of breast cancer and only one in ten of trained staff had superior knowledge to that found among a group of nursing auxiliaries. Personal experience was more influential than that gained professionally in affecting nurses' views (Knopf Elkind, 1981, 1982). In the context of cancer, this lack of knowledge may prevent nurses developing interpersonal skills precisely because their fears are similar to those of the lay public; 'getting close' to problems would lower their defences. 'Getting close' might also mean risking exposure of ignorance if difficult questions were asked. In addition to this, the giving of information about diagnosis and prognosis is often seen as the doctor's responsibility (Bond, 1978; McIntosh, 1974; Quint, 1972).

General Practitioners also find relating to patients with breast cancer difficult. The aims of their training have been to define and control disease, whereas breast cancer is situated at the limits of cultural control and scientific knowledge (Rosser and Maguire, 1982). Similarly, surgeons might feel distress for patients in part because of their own fears associated with breast cancer, but also because of the blamelessness of the victim, contrasting with diseases which might owe something to a patient's previous behaviour (Ray, 1981). Researchers are also vulnerable about cancer. Quint (1972, p.227), on undertaking a study of mastectomy patients, pointed out

> It was not just a matter of observer/reporter but of an active participant in a human engagement . . . we were caught in feelings of compassion . . . and we frequently suffered the anguish of wanting to do something.

This feeling of helplessness when witnessing suffering can be acute, even though the long-term goals of research are being kept in mind. My own experience and that of other research workers known to me is similar to that of Quint.

The Breast

Breasts have been cherished as the epitome of feminine charm, of a woman's sense of being intrinsically whole, and of sexual attractiveness and maternal adequacy over the years. Also they are constantly exploited for commercial gain and exhibited to sell anything and everything (Faulder, 1982). The permissive attitudes to nudity and sex disseminated by the media and to be seen in parts of our society can be constant reminders to us all of what it is that women have lost, or may lose. As a patient remarked 'I try to forget — but they are there every night — cleavages coming out at me from the box' (Tait and Maguire, 1981).

Amputation of the breast can pose such a threat to a woman's self-esteem and sense of sexual attractiveness that it can be a central issue in her psychological recovery (Witkin, 1978). Though three-quarters of a sample of nurses thought that such a threat might cause serious sexual problems for patients (Ray, 1984), two other studies suggest that nurses have limited knowledge of sexuality and that their conservative attitudes towards sex were related to this lack of knowledge (Payne, 1976; Fisher and Levin, 1983). The taboos and myths around the notion of sexuality are still present in many of those involved in care as well as in many patients, and as Webb (1984) writes, a nurse's supposedly holistic approach to care frequently ignores sexuality.

Public and Professional Controversy about Treatments

Anyone exposed to media reporting is likely to have noticed the arguments regarding the efficacy of treatments for breast cancer, and whether they are worth the unpleasant side effects that many of them produce. Consequently, many of the lay public, patients included, know more about these controversies than those involved in care. Another difficulty concerns the speed with which medical practice is changing. Many of the research findings reported in this chapter occurred when nine out of ten doctors performed a mastectomy for early breast cancer. Now only about five out of ten doctors do so: the rest are likely to perform a partial removal of the breast (*The Guardian*, 1984). This flight to conservative surgery, based on so few clinical trials, may well be a response to public pressure backed by a considerable amount of research on the psychological impact of mastectomy. When admitting that knowledge about the physical process of breast cancer was limited, Denton and Baum (1983) wrote that improved quality of care was within our grasp because of the research into quality-of-life issues. But do patients agree?

The Patient as Health Service Consumer

Certainly, many patients are looking for ways of improving their quality of life, but increasingly some see this as only possible through their own efforts. It is not only in the USA that the waves of consumerism are washing the shores of medical practice and women are establishing their beachhead (Schain, 1980). The trend towards self-help in alternative therapies continues. Simonton and Simonton (1978), Kidman (1983) and Faulder (1984) ask how it is that we know so little about the clinical trials for breast cancer treatments that so clearly could affect us, when true informed consent should be our goal.

Issues Concerning the Care of Patients with Breast Cancer

This broader context into which issues about breast cancer must fit presents a challenge to nurses who wish to develop good interpersonal skills. They will not only need flexibility and knowledge to accommodate these changes occurring in attitudes and practice, but they will also need to influence those with and for whom they work, so that they understand and support them. Without this, good communication is difficult.

The Psychological Effects of Breast Cancer and its Treatments

Research findings are extensive in this field, from descriptive studies affording useful insights to a few randomised and controlled studies from which generalisations can be made. Of these, two British studies produced broadly similar findings. Maguire *et al.* (1978a) found that 25 per cent of patients needed treatment for anxiety and depression, compared with 10 per cent in a control group; also 33 per cent experienced moderate to severe sexual difficulties compared with 8 per cent in the control group: these difficulties were apparent one year after mastectomy. Similarly, Morris, Green and White (1977) found that 23 per cent of patients were moderately to severely depressed two years after mastectomy, compared with 10 per cent in a control group: importantly, 33 per cent of the experimental group were dissatisfied with the information they received. In the USA, Worden and Weisman (1977) found that about 20 per cent of women were depressed at the end of the year following mastectomy. Having breast cancer and mastectomy is clearly traumatic for about 20 to 30 per cent of women. When one considers what a large number even those percentages entail, that is a great deal of suffering (Graydon 1982).

Problems in Communication

In her review of the literature on the psychological effects of breast cancer and its treatments, Morris (1979) concluded that for the one third of the total number of women who were not able, psychologically, to resume their former life style, their *problems would be unlikely to be detected by those treating them and might remain unresolved.*

The proliferation of studies revealing inadequate communications with patients having breast cancer points to the size of the problem. Bond (1982) cites several studies in her review on communications in cancer nursing. Maguire (1976) found that only a quarter of distressed women mentioned this to the clinic surgeon though many showed their upset, non-verbally. The surgeons only responded to 5 per cent of these cues directly and when they did so the women's anxiety decreased. These problems were not confined to clinics. Maguire also noted that only one in twenty interactions with patients on a ward were concerned with the patients' emotional well-being. Woods and Earp (1978) found that women were not prepared for post-operative experiences, and several authors have observed that discussion of emotional problems did not occur at the times of maximum emotional stress, if at all (Jamison, Wellisch and Pasnau, 1978; Pfefferbaum, Pasnau, Jamison and Wellisch, 1977; Quint, 1963; Wellisch, Jamison and Pasnau, 1978). Problems of inconsistent information arose partly because of the variety of doctors that patients met at follow-up, due to the rotational system (Tait, Maguire and Brooke, 1980), but also because patients tended to rely on each other for information and as an outlet for emotional problems. Consequently, they had many misconceptions (Bond, 1978).

Recent studies do not give us cause for complacency. Silberfarb, Maurer and Crowthorne (1980a) found that though one-third of their sample had sexual problems, these were 'sadly neglected'. In Feeley, Peel and Devlin's (1982) study, one-quarter of the sample felt they had inadequate information pre-operatively, and 13 of them claimed that they were unaware of the likelihood of mastectomy. As with Downie's (1976) research, communication about prostheses provision was inadequate. It is not surprising, therefore, that Bullough (1981) found that only 20 per cent of patients could identify a nurse as a significant source of information, and only 25 per cent identified her as a source of emotional support.

There are also difficulties in communicating about specific toxic treatments. Maguire (1976) noted that, as at other stages of treatment, very little of the distress patients experienced with radiotherapy was detected by nurses or doctors. These findings are in line with Mitchell and Glicksman's (1977) findings, which showed that 82 per cent of patients felt that neither their physician nor radiotherapist could help with emotional problems, and 52 per cent felt that their referring physician had not prepared them in any way for the experience of radiotherapy. Silberfarb *et al.* (1980a) noted that women receiving radiotherapy showed significantly more distress than those not receiving treatment, and they showed this by making 'unsolicited and negative comments'. Gyllenskold (1982), used a psychodynamic frame of reference to describe and interpret her observations of women with breast cancer, and showed how women found radiotherapy eerie and frightening — yet pretended they had no problems. Such pretence consumed their already depleted energy, so it was of great value to the women to have the chance to voice their concerns.

The toxicity of chemotherapy for breast cancer is described by Meyerowitz, Sparks and Spears (1979) in terms of increased disruption and emotional stress. However, Silberfarb, Philibert and Levine (1980b) found it was possible for patients and those involved in care to have unrealistic views of the patients' true emotional state because of the significant relationship between cognitive impairment and chemotherapy. Maguire *et al.* (1980a) showed that only a minority of women reported the toxicity they experienced to those concerned with care, though this was in part due to lack of probing by clinic staff. Unfortunately, there was a strong link between this non-disclosure and the failure of these women to complete what might be a life-saving treatment.

The impact of this failure to communicate has been movingly described by those with advanced breast cancer (Flynn, 1977; Kaplan, 1983). The latter wrote that the prospect of abandonment by loved ones, friends and health care professionals was more fearful than the prospect of dying. These findings are similar to those reflecting dissatisfaction at a general level in doctor-patient communications (Ley, 1977; Maguire, 1981) and in nurse-patient communications (Faulkner, 1979; Macleod Clark, 1981).

Additional Reasons for Poor Communication. In addition to those reasons raised by discussion of the broader context of breast cancer, Maguire (1978) and Maguire, Tait and Brooke (1980b) have suggested that patients perceived nurses as busy, and mainly interested in their physical well-being. The patients did not want to be labelled as inadequate or uncooperative, and wanted to protect the staff from strain.

Both patients and nurses often doubted if anything could be done to improve the patients' situation. Nurses worried that it was intrusive to ask patients about their feelings, and even obvious problems were thought to be understandable and so were disregarded. Also, these kinds of questions about emotional issues were too time-consuming, and nurses were not trained in the relevant skills. My own experience in teaching nurses communication skills has shown that these objections are still being raised, though in many cases, because 'communication skills' are more fashionable now, nurses say the most inhibiting factor for them is their felt lack of knowledge about the breast disease process, its treatments, and what can be done about various problems.

Common Statements About the Importance of Communication/ Interpersonal Skills. Though it is clear that nurses are in part responsible for many of the problems relating to poor communication, the paradox is that many nurses who write about nursing patients with breast disease either explicitly or implicitly emphasise the need for good practice in this field. Some cite the importance of their previous experience as patients in heightening consciousness about the problem (Barbour, 1975; Coburn, 1975; Cox, 1979; Kennerly, 1977). (Though this common experience of having been a patient with breast disease does enable formation of a special bond, my discussions with several nurses in this situation leads me to believe that it can also be a great strain on ex-patient nurses to watch the effects of toxic treatments or advancing disease — more threatening perhaps than to a nurse who has not had breast cancer.)

Care studies stress the importance of 'emotional support' at an anecdotal level but do not show how this may be accomplished (Armstrong, 1980; Noe, 1980; Roberts, 1975). The information needs of patients are stressed by both Moetzinger and Dauber (1982) and Warren (1979) regarding chemotherapy, and Rutledge (1982) about breast reconstruction. Patient education and support programmes by health care professionals, and in some cases ex-patients as volunteers, are advocated by many people (Bloom, Ross and Burnell, 1978; Farash, 1979; Ferlic, Goldman and Kennedy, 1979; Miller and Nygren, 1978; Reynolds, Sachs, Davis and Hall, 1981; Sachs *et al.*, 1981; Schain, 1976; Schmidt, Kiss and Hibbert, 1974; Spiegel, Bloom and Yalom, 1981: Vachon and Lyall, 1976). Programmes promoting patients' rehabilitation, by information and communication with ex-patients, have been described by Kleinman, Mantell and Alexander (1977) who reported on group work, and by Lasser and Clarke (1972) who reported working on an individual basis.

The importance of communication, assessment or counselling skills is acknowledged in several descriptions of the specialist nurse's role in breast care (Baum and Jones, 1979; Denton, 1981; Denton and Baum, 1983; Maguire *et al.*, 1980b; Osborne, 1978; Tait *et al.*, 1980, 1982; Thomson, 1983; Wilbur, 1983).

Evaluation of Specific Intervention Schemes

The specialist nurse studies quoted demonstrate interest and enthusiasm for good interpersonal skills in achieving rehabilitation of patients; however, only two studies give details of the training and methods used to achieve good communication (Maguire *et al.*, 1980c; Tait *et al.*, 1982). Of prime importance is the fact that very few intervention schemes have been evaluated. Watson (1983), in a review of the literature on evaluated psychosocial interventions with cancer patients, found that it was difficult to draw conclusions about the comparative benefits of group or individual rehabilitation programmes. It did seem clear, though, that the need for help continued beyond the initial period of diagnosis. Maguire *et al.* (1980d) and Maguire (1984) indicated that until predictors of vulnerability were reliably established, monitoring of the patients' emotional state was advisable, and for some patients support and therapy would be required over time.

Work on Evaluating Group Interventions

Encouraging findings have been reported by several researchers (Bloom *et al.*, 1978; Farash, 1979; Miller and Nygren, 1978; Reynolds *et al.*, 1981; Sachs *et al.*, 1981; Vachon and Lyall, 1976; Winnick and Robbins, 1977). Two controlled studies, Ferlic *et al.* (1979) and Spiegel *et al.* (1981), found significant improvements for those in counselled groups.

Work on Evaluating Individual Nursing Interventions

This area of work can present difficulties — such as whether findings are generalisable given the very different contexts in which nursing care has been given. However, relative to other specialist nursing areas, such as stoma care, where evaluation of the nursing contribution is in its infancy, evaluation of various schemes concerning breast care is well advanced.

A controlled study in Wales (Baum and Jones, 1979) showed that a pre-operative group of mastectomy patients counselled by a nurse showed lower state-anxiety scores than a group receiving routine care. However, there were no immediate post-operative differences and longer term follow-up has not been reported. Another controlled study in the USA (Gordon *et al.*, 1980) evaluated the effects of a psychosocial rehabilitation programme on patients with melanoma, breast and lung cancers. A psychiatric nurse, social workers and psychologists worked as oncology counsellors on a one-to-one basis with patients. Results showed that the counselled group had a more rapid decline of anxiety and hostility, a more realistic outlook on life, a greater number of patients returning to work and more active use of time. A further controlled study was set up in England by Maguire *et al.* (1980d) to determine if counselling by a specialist nurse might prevent the psychiatric morbidity associated with breast cancer. The results of this trial showed that counselling failed to prevent morbidity. However, regular monitoring of the women's progress led the nurse to recognise and refer 76 per cent of those who needed psychiatric help. Only 15 per cent of the control group who warranted help were recognised or referred. Consequently, 12 to 18 months after mastectomy there was much less psychiatric morbidity in the counselled group (12 per cent) than in the control group (39 per cent).

The effect of this same counselling on the physical disability and social recovery of patients was also evaluated. 12 to 18 months following mastectomy, those helped by the nurse showed a greater social recovery, return to work, adaptation to breast loss and satisfaction with their breast prosthesis. The nurse had little impact on physical disability (Maguire *et al.*, 1983). A cost benefit study was also undertaken on this project (Maguire *et al.*, 1982) which showed that a specialist nurse service could be implemented at little extra cost to the NHS, because of savings made in patient care.

Because of the relative success of this specialist nurse project, the DHSS funded a study to determine if ward and community nurses given similar training could be as effective as the specialist nurse. The study also aimed to determine if specialist nurses could be as successful if they limited their contact to one home visit, and put the onus on the patient to initiate subsequent contact (Wilkinson *et al.*, 1983). The training of the ward nurses and the results of that training are reported by Faulkner and Maguire (1984). Preliminary results have suggested that the training was effective with ward staff, and that limited contact by the specialist nurse was as successful as regular monitoring. If these results hold in the final analysis, specialist nurses could be released from some of their routine monitoring of patients and would be able to develop a resource nurse role, teaching interviewing and assessment skills to those routinely involved in care and accepting referrals of special cases.

Data have been collected, but not yet analysed, for two other research studies. One, in London, is a controlled trial looking at the effect of counselling by a specialist nurse on patients' ability to cope, following mastectomy. The other is a collaborative study between Edinburgh and London nursing research centres. It looks at the aftercare of the mastectomy patients, and if (and how) general nurses and clinical nurse specialists aid patients' adjustment.

The Training of the Specialist Nurse in Breast Care

This was a crucial factor in the relative success of the specialist nurse project (Maguire *et al.*, 1980a, 1983). A non-psychiatric nurse was chosen to see if she could be taught the skills necessary to elicit social and psychiatric problems. The training took 3 months and consisted of:

(1) knowledge of breast cancer, its treatments and their physical, psychological and social sequelae;

(2) appreciation of differing approaches to aftercare;

(3) knowledge of the range and provision of breast prostheses and clothing;

(4) identification of resources and appreciation of their utilisation;

(5) essential interviewing skills;

(6) the topics necessary for assessment, and the repertoire of questions needed to elicit social and psychiatric problems.

The Theoretical Interview

The initial hypothesis of Maguire's specialist nurse project was that the nurse might prevent psychiatric morbidity in patients. So, it was hoped that the nurse might provide a psychotherapeutic medium for change. In a theoretical description of the interview, based on Rogerian concepts (Rogers, 1942, 1951), it was stated that the purpose of the interview should be (Bernstein and Dana, 1970):

(1) to establish the relationship between health care professional and patient (in this, the value and dignity of the individual were respected so that with the professional's assistance the patient could find adjustment and meaning in her life);

(2) to elicit information about the patient's condition;

(3) to permit observation of the patient's behaviour.

A particular facet of the skills required concerned the importance of accepting and reflecting feelings, but an unstructured approach was advocated. These principles have formed the basis of many counselling courses.

Interviewing Skills

Maguire's approach to teaching interviewing and assessment skills was pragmatic and directive. The time-honoured apprenticeship system was ineffective, so systematic feedback was given on audiotaped interviews. Such feedback on performance has proved effective in helping medical students acquire similar skills (Maguire *et al.*, 1978b). Particular attention was paid to helping the nurse recognise the many verbal and non-verbal clues that patients gave about their problems. Deficiencies in these skills were similar to those revealed by medical students (Maguire and Rutter 1976). The nurse also needed to know how to control an interview, that is, how to encourage patients to keep to the point without alienating them. The tendency of the nurse to reassure patients before she had clarified what they were really worried about, and to jolly them along, had to be countered. (This method of feedback by audiotape provides a relatively cheap and simple way to manage self-assessment once the principles of interviewing skills have been learnt. As the specialist nurse for most of Maguire's project and holding subjective views on my own skills, I have found it a salutary experience to hear how my actual performance rated against the specific criteria developed by Maguire. Other nurses using this method suggest that they have had similar experiences).

Identification of Patients' Problems: The Use of a Standardised Assessment

Previous research has identified the problems commonly experienced by patients and the factors that predict a less favourable psychological and social outcome. These topics were included in the assessment, not only to enable detection of problems, but also to persuade patients that it was legitimate to talk about them. The nurse therefore focused on monitoring the patient's state, identifying problems and assessing the patient's coping capacity, rather than 'counselling'. Even with this apparently limited approach patients would say how helpful it was to be able to talk about their problems once assessment was made. Many problems could be helped immediately, others required referral from the nurse.

The topics covered included:

(1) reactions to breast disease;
(2) previous experience of cancer;
(3) reaction to mastectomy;
(4) other stresses and difficulties;
(5) interpersonal relationships and;
(6) psychological reaction.

A repertoire of questions to identify concerns was learnt, and this was especially important in the probes necessary to elicit an anxiety state or depressive illness. These derived from a standardised psychiatric interview (Wing, Cooper and Sartorious, 1974). For the DHSS funded project on specialist, ward and community nurse comparisons of counselling, these necessary topics and questions were developed into manuals that could be used in conjunction with the standardised assessment forms (Tait *et al.*, 1982).

Factors That Predicted a Less Favourable Outcome

Empirical investigations have shown certain factors are either liable to result in individual breakdown or are protective against breakdown under stress. Adequate social support has been shown to be important as a protective factor. Brown and Harris (1978) identified the importance of one factor in particular that made women more likely to experience depressive breakdown following a 'severe life-event' (such as mastectomy), namely the lack of someone in whom a woman could confide and who understood her — a 'confiding tie'.

Recently Maguire and van Dam (1983) found that the presence of a 'confiding tie' had a protective effect against later development of depressive illness or sexual problems. This, in itself, makes a good case for the nurse to become the confiding tie in the crisis stages, at least for patients who have no-one else. Other predictors of vulnerability were dread of mastectomy, and depression. Denton and Baum (1982) showed that fear of mutilation as a prime pre-operative concern was strongly associated with later psychiatric referral. Following surgery, Maguire found that development of moderate to severe pain, swelling in the affected arm, toxicity due to chemotherapy and failure to adapt to breast loss were predictive of psychiatric problems. Bloom (1982) and Northouse (1981) also showed how perceived social support could help patients' adjustment.

If these findings can be replicated, nurses could restrict their attention to those most likely to develop problems. However, that hope is founded on the assumption that nurses would base their practice on research findings. There is evidence that this does not always happen (Hunt, 1981)!

Referral Procedures

A feature of Maguire's specialist nurse study was that the nurse used a direct referral procedure to psychiatry. When describing the problems I had experienced and the help I had received in this study (Tait *et al.*, 1980), I wrote about the difficulties experienced by patients, and those involved in care, concerning the stigma of psychiatry; I also mentioned the fact that in many cases the medical teams did not believe that patients required psychiatric help. This question of the difficulty nurses may have regarding referral procedures has been raised by Breckman (1983). Traditionally, the power of referral within the NHS has been with general practitioners or consultants — but nurses have carried out certain referrals by custom (e.g. to social workers or dieticians). But is the detection of emotional illness a medical or a nursing responsibility? Another issue relates to the willingness, or otherwise, of psychiatrists to interest themselves in the stresses that women with breast cancer experience. Many nurses in breast cancer care suggest that there is no one to refer to. However, this may be a chicken-and-egg situation, and motivated nurses who can accurately identify emotional illness should be able to put adequate pressure on those professionals who could help. They would have evidence from research studies to support their arguments.

The Nurse's Need for Support

The acknowledgement of this need has already been made. In Maguire's specialist nurse study he anticipated that support would be required for the nurse, and provided it. The nature of the work, based on a process approach, meant that as the nurse, I knew some patients well, felt close to them and consequently suffered when they did. It has been realised that the nurse's availability to patients over a period of time (one year) might be in their interests: they are known to be particularly at risk three months post-operatively (Maguire *et al.*, 1980a; Weisman and Worden, 1976). Without support, I am not sure that I would have finished the project. On the other hand, what is rarely mentioned is the potential for personal growth that exists when privileged to observe how resourceful and courageous many patients are. However, this development of the nurse is only likely to occur if she feels understood and supported. Faulkner (1984) writes that expecting nurses to use a process approach without realisation of the implications, such as need for knowledge, or health education, need for communication skills and need for support, is unrealistic. Research on support for nurses is minimal. Vachon *et al.* (1978) showed it to be important and Yasko (1983) showed that a greater degree of 'burnout' was experienced by those who did not receive adequate support at work, among other factors.

Development of the Specialist/Resource Nurse in Breast Care

The findings outlined in this chapter perhaps raise more questions than they answer. Many patients with breast cancer, whether in future they do or do not have a mastectomy, are likely to need careful monitoring at least for the first three months post-operatively, and at times of disease recurrence (Silberfarb *et al.*, 1980a). The question is, who can and who will do this? Perhaps hospital and community nurses can be taught the essential skills, but they are unlikely to see such work as a priority unless given access to knowledgeable advice, support and encouragement. On present evidence they will not receive much support from general practitioners (Rosser and Maguire, 1982). Part of their motivation might come from a specialist resource nurse, who would also be available to accept referrals from nurses as well as others. Though this kind of nurse is rare, in a recent study most nurses in the sample felt that a specialist nurse was the correct person to counsel breast cancer patients (Ray, 1984).

There has been a gradual increase in the numbers of breast care specialist nurses since the mid 1970s, and there are now approximately 30 of them working in the United Kingdom. Some have joint appointments as stoma care nurses. These breast care nurses have emerged on an *ad hoc* basis, based mainly in nursing, with a few funded by medical budgets or research grants. Their job specifications vary as does their training. Though several nurses have been on counselling courses and found them helpful, very few have had training in interviewing and assessment skills as described in this chapter. It does seem as though identification of a patient's problems by these skills is a prerequisite to counselling, which might then enable the patient to help herself. There is now a Breast Care Forum, started in 1983 and included within the RCN Oncology Nursing Society. This should provide the opportunity for development of a relevant training course — but, as Maguire asked in (1980b), will nurses grasp this nettle?

Most of the women who have breast cancer are treated in district general hospitals and are unlikely to have contact with specialist doctors or nurses on a breast unit. Although some of these women may use voluntary organisations such as the Mastectomy Association for practical advice and support, many will have problems that are neglected. They could be helped by nurses routinely involved in care, if, in addition to being motivated, using communication skills and knowing where to get advice, nurses understand that having breast cancer is often a process and not an event, therefore interventions may be needed over a long period. Also, that patients' behaviours and attitudes do not just reside 'objectively' in patients, but are in part constructed by those with whom patients interact. The way nurses may define patients' behaviour, and thus react, can be the product of their own fears and anxieties because of the emotive context of breast cancer. If nurses can allow these concerns to surface, be accepted, and themselves feel supported, interpersonal skills are likely to improve.

References

Armstrong, K. (1980) 'Mastectomy: One day at a time', *Nursing Mirror*, 10 January, 20-1

Barbour, T. (1975) 'I Travelled the Mastectomy Road', *Supervisor Nurse*, 75, 40-3

Baum, M. (1981) *Breast Cancer. The Facts*, Oxford University Press: Oxford

Baum, M. and Jones, I. (1979) 'Mastectomy: Counselling removes patients' fears', *Nursing Mirror*, 8 March, 38-40

Bernstein, L. and Dana, R. (1970) *Interviewing and the Health Professions*, Appleton Century Crofts: New York

Bloom, J. (1982) 'Social Support: Accommodation to Stress and Adjustment to Breast Cancer', *Social Science and Medicine, 16,* 1329-38

Bloom, J.R., Ross, R.D. and Burnell, G. (1978), 'The Effect of Social Support on Patient Adjustment After Breast Surgery', *Patient Counselling and Health Education*, Autumn, 50-9

Bond, S. (1978) 'Processes of Communication About Cancer in a Radiotherapy Department' unpublished Ph. D. thesis: University of Edinburgh

Bond, S. (1982) 'Communications in Cancer Nursing' in M.C. Cahoon (ed.) *Cancer Nursing*, Churchill Livingstone: Edinburgh

Breckman, B. (1983) 'Referrals: Whose problem, whose responsibility?, *Nursing Times*, 19 October, 58-60

Brown, G.W. and Harris, T. (1978) *The Social Origins of Depression*, Tavistock: London

Bullough, B. (1981) 'Nurses as Teachers and Support Persons for Breast Cancer Patients', *Cancer Nursing*, 4, 221-30

Coburn, D. (1975) 'Anticipating Breast Surgery', *American Journal of Nursing*, 75, 1483-5

Comaroff, J. and Maguire, P. (1981) 'Ambiguity and the Search for Meaning. Childhood Leukaemia in the Modern Clinical Context', *Social Science and Medicine, 15B*, 115-23

Cox, J. (1979) 'Breast Tumour: Taking the patient's point of view', *Nursing Mirror*, 22 March, 47-8

Davison, R.L. (1965) 'Opinion of Nurses on Cancer: Its treatment and curability. A survey among nurses in the public health service', *British Journal of Preventive Medicine, 19*, 24-9

Denton, S. (1981) 'The Role of the Nurse Counsellor' in M. Baum (ed.) *Breast Cancer. The Facts*, Oxford University Press: Oxford

Denton, S. and Baum, M. (1982) 'Can we Predict Which Women Will Fail to Cope with Mastectomy?', *Clinical Oncology*, 8, 375-9

Denton, S. and Baum, M. (1983) 'Psychological Aspects of Breast Cancer' in R. Margalese (ed.), *Breast Cancer*, Churchill Livingstone: Edinburgh

Downie, P.A. (1976) 'Post-Mastectomy Survey', *Nursing Mirror*, 25 March, 65-6

Farash, J. (1979) 'Effect of Counselling on Resolution of Loss and Body Image Disturbance Following Mastectomy', *Dissertation Abstracts International*, 39, 4027

Faulder, C. (1982) *Breast Cancer. A Guide to its Early Detection*, Virago: London

Faulder, C. (1984) 'A Conspiracy of Silence: When your treatment is on trial', *Good Housekeeping*, February, p.54

Faulkner, A. (1979) 'Monitoring Nurse-Patient Conversation on a Ward', *Nursing Times*, 30 August, Occasional Paper

Faulkner, A. (1984) 'Health Education and Nursing', *Nursing Times*, 29 February, 45-6

Faulkner, A. and Maguire, P. (1984) 'Teaching Assessment Skills' in A. Faulkner (ed.) *Recent Advances in Nursing*, 7, *Communication*, Churchill Livingstone: Edinburgh

Feeley, T.M., Peel, A.L.G. and Devlin, H.B. (1982) 'Mastectomy and its Consequences', *British Medical Journal*, *284*, 1246

Ferlic, M., Goldman, A. and Kennedy, B.J. (1979) 'Group Counselling in Adult patients with Advanced Cancer', *Cancer*, *43*, 760-6

Fisher, S. and Levin, D. (1983) 'The Sexual Knowledge and Attitudes of Professional Nurses Caring for Oncology Patients', *Cancer Nursing*, *6*, 55-61

Flynn, E. (1977) 'What it Means to Battle Against Cancer', *American Journal of Nursing*, *77*, 261-2

Gordon, W., Friedenbergs, I., Diller, L., Hibbard, M., Wolfe, C., Levine, L., Lipkins, R., Ezraeki, O. and Lucido, D. (1980) 'Efficacy of Psychosocial Intervention with Cancer Patients', *Journal of Consulting and Clinical Psychology*, *48*, 743-59

Graydon, J. (1982) 'Aspects of Breast Cancer' in M.C. Cahoon (ed.), *Cancer Nursing*, Churchill Livingstone: Edinburgh

Guardian, The (1984) 'A Cautious Optimism' (by Liz Grint) 25 January, p.9

Gyllenskold, K. (1982) *Breast Cancer: The Psychological Effects of the Disease and its Treatment*, Tavistock: London

Hunt, J. (1981) 'Indications for Nursing Practice: The use of research findings,' *Journal of Advanced Nursing*, *6*, 189-94

Jamison, K.R., Wellisch, D.K., Pasnau, R.O.E. (1978) 'Psychosocial Aspects of Mastectomy: The woman's perspective', *American Journal of Psychiatry*, *135*, 432-6

Kaplan, M. (1983) 'Viewpoint: The cancer patient', *Cancer Nursing*, *6*, 103-7

Kennerley, S.F. (1977) 'What I've Learned about Mastectomy', *American Journal of Nursing*, *77*, 1430-1437

Kidman, B. (1983) *A Gentle Way with Cancer*, Century: Aylesbury, Bucks.

Kleinman, M., Mantell, J. and Alexander, E. (1977) 'R After Social Death: The cancer patient as counsellor', *Community Mental Health Journal*, *13*, 115-23

Knopf Elkind, A. (1981) 'The Accuracy of Nurses' Knowledge of Survival Rates for Early Cancer in Four Sites', *Journal of Advanced Nursing*, *6*, 35-40

Knopf Elkind, A. (1982) 'Nurses' Views About Cancer', *Journal of Advanced Nursing*, *7*, 43-50

Lasser, T. and Clarke, W. (1972) *Reach to Recovery*, Simon and Schuster: New York

Ley, P. (1977) 'Psychological Studies of Doctor-Patient Communication' in S. Rachman (ed.), *Contributions to Medical Psychology*, *1*, Pergamon: Oxford

Macleod Clark, J. (1981) 'Communication in Nursing: Analysing nurse-patient conversations', *Nursing Times*, *77*, 12-18

Maguire, P. (1976) 'The Psychological and Social Sequelae of Mastectomy' in J.G. Howells (ed.) *Modern Perspectives in the Psychiatric Aspects of Surgery*, Churchill Livingstone: Edinburgh

Maguire, P. (1978) 'The Psychological Effects of Cancers and Their Treatments' in R. Tiffany (ed.), *Oncology for Nurses and Health Care Professionals*, *2*, *Care and Support*, Allen and Unwin: London

Maguire, P. (1981) 'Doctor-Patient Skills' in M. Argyle (ed.) *Social Skills and Health*, Methuen: London

Maguire, P. (1984) 'Psychological Reactions to Breast Cancer and its Treatment' in G. Bonnadonna (ed.) *Breast Cancer, Diagnosis and Management*, Wiley: Chichester

Maguire, P. and Rutter, D. (1976) 'Training Medical Students to Communicate' in A. Bennett (ed.) *Communication Between Doctors and Patients*, Oxford University Press: Oxford

Maguire, P. and van Dam, F. (1983) 'Psychological Aspects of Breast Cancer: Workshop report', *European Journal Cancer Clinical Oncology*, *19*, 1735-40

Maguire, P., Brooke, M., Tait, A., Thomas, C. and Sellwood, R. (1983) 'The Effect of Counselling on Physical Disability and Social Recovery After Mastectomy', *Clinical Oncology*, *9*, 319-24

Maguire, P., Lee, E.G., Bevington, D.J., Kuchemann, C., Crabtree, R.J. and Cornell, C.E. (1978a) 'Psychiatric Problems in the First Year after Mastectomy', *British Medical Journal, 1,* 963-965

Maguire, P., Pentol, A., Allen, D., Tait, A., Brooke, M., and Sellwood, R. (1982) 'Cost of Counselling Women Who Undergo Mastectomy', *British Medical Journal, 284,* 1933-5

Maguire, P., Roe, P., Goldberg, D., Jones, S., Hyde, C. and O'Dowd, T. (1978b) 'The Value of Feedback in Teaching Interviewing Skills to Medical Students', *Psychological Medicine, 8,* 695-704

Maguire, P., Tait, A., Brooke, M., Thomas, C., Howat, J. and Sellwood, R. (1980a) 'Psychiatric Morbidity and Physical Toxicity Associated with Mastectomy', *British Medical Journal, 281,* 1176-9

Maguire, P., Tait, A. and Brooke, M. (1980b) 'Emotional Aspects of Mastectomy — A conspiracy of pretence', *Nursing Mirror,* 10 January, 17-19

Maguire, P., Tait, A., Brooke, M. and Sellwood, R. (1980c) 'Mastectomy: Planning a caring programme', *Nursing Mirror,* 17 January, 35-7

Maguire, P., Tait, A., Brooke, M., Thomas, C. and Sellwood, R. (1980d) 'Effect of Counselling on the Psychiatric Morbidity Associated with Mastectomy', *British Medical Journal ,2,* 1454-6

Mastrovito, C. (1972) 'Emotional Considerations in Cancer and Stroke', *New York State Journal of Medicine, 72,* 2874-7

McIntosh, J. (1974) 'Processes of Communication, Information Seeking and Control Associated with Cancer: A selective review of the literature', *Social Science and Medicine, 9,* 167-87

Meyerowitz, B., Sparks, R. and Spears, I. (1979) 'Adjuvant Chemotherapy for Breast Carcinoma : Psychosocial implications', *Cancer, 43,* 1613-8

Miller, M.W. and Nygren, C. (1978) 'Living With Cancer: Coping behaviours', *Cancer Nursing, 1,* 297-302

Mitchell, G. and Glicksman, A. (1977) 'Cancer Patients: Knowledge and attitudes', *Cancer, 40,* 61-6

Moetzinger, C. and Dauber, L.G. (1982) 'The Management of the Patient with Breast Cancer', *Cancer Nursing, 5,* 287-91

Morris, T. (1979) 'Psychological Adjustment to Mastectomy', *Cancer Treatment Reviews, 6,* 41-61

Morris, T., Green, S. and White, P. (1977) 'Psychological and Social Adjustment to Mastectomy', *Cancer, 40,* 2381-7

Noe, B. (1980) 'A Time for Reassurance', *Nursing Mirror, 150,* 40-1

Northouse, L.L. (1981) 'Mastectomy Patients and Fear of Cancer Recurrence', *Cancer Nursing, 4,* 213-20

O'Brien, J. (1978) 'Mirror, mirror, why me?' *Nursing Mirror,* 36-7

Osborne, S. (1978) 'The Role of the Specialist Nurse in the Breast Unit', *Nursing Times, 74,* 1201-2

Payne, T. (1976) 'Sexuality of Nurses: Correlations of knowledge, attitudes and behaviour', *Nursing Research, 25,* 286-92

Pfefferbaum, B., Pasnau, R., Jamison, K. and Wellisch, D., (1977) 'A Comprehensive Program of Psychosocial Care for Mastectomy Patients', *International Journal of Psychiatry in Medicine, 8,* 63-72

Quint, J.C. (1963) 'Mastectomy — Symbol of Cure or Warning Sign?', *General Practitioner, XXIX,* 119-24

Quint, J.C. (1972) 'Institutionalised Practices of Information Control', in E. Freidson and J. Lorber (eds.), *Medical Men and Their Work: A Sociological Reader,* Aldine Atherton: Chicago

Ray, C. (1981) *Perspectives on Cancer: The surgeon's viewpoint,* Paper delivered to the Conference of the Social Psychology Section of British Psychological Society

Ray, C. (1984) 'Nurses' Perceptions of Early Breast Cancer and Mastectomy and their Psychological Implications and of the Role of Health Professionals in Providing Support', *International Journal of Nursing Studies, 21*, 101-10

Reynolds, S., Sachs, S., Davis, J. and Hall, P. (1981) 'Meeting the Information Needs of Patients on Clinical Trials: A new approach', *Cancer Nursing, 4*, 227-30

Roberts, J. (1975) 'Mastectomy — A patient's point of view', *Nursing Times, 71*, 1290-1

Rogers, C.R. (1942) *Counselling and Psychotherapy*, Houghton Mifflin: Boston

Rogers, C.R. (1951) *Client Centered Therapy*, Houghton Mifflin: Boston

Rosser, J. and Maguire, P. (1982) 'Dilemmas in General Practice: The care of the cancer patient', *Social Science and Medicine, 16*, 315-22

Rutledge, D.N. (1982) 'A Nurse's Knowledge of Breast Reconstruction: A catalyst for earlier treatment of breast cancer', *Cancer Nursing, 5*, 469-73

Sachs, S.H., Davis, J.M., Reynolds, S.A., Spagnola, M., Hall, P. and Bloch, A. (1981) 'Comparative Results of Post-Mastectomy Rehabilitation in a Specialised and a Community Hospital', *Cancer, 48*, 1251

Schain, W. (1976) 'Psychosocial Issues in Counselling Mastectomy Patients', *The Counselling Psychologist, 6*, 45-9

Schain, W. (1980) 'Patients' Rights in Decision Making: The case for personalism versus paternalism in health care', *Cancer, 46*, 1035-41

Schmidt, W., Kiss, M. and Hibbert, L. (1974) 'The Team Approach to Rehabilitation After Mastectomy', *American Operating-room Nurse Journal, 4*, 821-36

Silberfarb, P.M., Maurer, L.H., and Crowthorne, C.S. (1980a) 'Psychosocial Aspects of Neoplastic Disease: I, Functional status of breast cancer patients during different treatment regimes', *American Journal of Psychiatry, 136*, 450-5

Silberfarb, P.M., Philibert, D. and Levine, P. (1980b) 'Psychosocial Aspects of Neoplastic Disease: II, Affective and cognitive effects of chemotherapy in cancer patients', *American Journal of Psychiatry, 137*, 597-601

Simonton, C. and Simonton, S. (1978) *Getting Well Again*, Bantam: London

Sontag, S. (1979) *Illness as Metaphor*, Allen Lane: London

Speigel, D., Bloom, J. and Yalom, I. (1981) 'Group Support for Patients with Metastatic Cancer', *Archives of General Psychiatry, 38*, 527

Tait, A. and Maguire, P. (1981) *Patients' Perceptions of Breast Cancer*, Paper delivered to the Conference of the Social Psychology Section of British Psychological Society

Tait, A. Maguire, P. and Brooke, M. (1980) 'Plan into Practice', *Nursing Mirror, 150*, 19-21

Tait, A., Maguire, P., Faulkner, A., Brooke, M., Wilkinson, S., Thomson, L. and Sellwood, R. (1982) 'Improving Communication Skills: Use of a semi-structured assessment following mastectomy', *Nursing Times*, 22 December, 2181-4

Thomson, L. (1983) *The Specialist Nurse as Resource and Practitioner*, Paper delivered to the Nursing Section of European Congress of Clinical Oncology, November

Vachon, M.L.S. and Lyall. W.A.L. (1976) 'Applying Psychiatric Techniques to Patients with Cancer', *Hospital and Community Psychiatry, 27*, 582-4

Vachon, M.L.S. and Lyall, W.A.L. (1976) 'Applying Psychiatric Techniques to Management of Stress in Health Professionals Working with Advanced Cancer Patients', *Death Education, 1*, 365-75

Warren, B. (1979) 'Adjuvant Chemotherapy for Breast Disease: The nurse's role', *Cancer Nursing, 2*, 32-4

Watson, M. (1983) 'Psychosocial Intervention with Cancer Patients: A review', *Psychosocial Medicine, 13*, 839-46

Webb, C. (1984) 'How would you feel?' *Nursing Times, Community Outlook*, February, 27-8

184 *Issues Arising from Mastectomy Nursing*

Weisman, A.D. (1979) *Coping with Cancer*, McGraw Hill: New York

Weisman, A.D. and Worden, J. (1976) 'The Existential Plight in Cancer: Significance of first 100 days', *International Journal of Psychiatry in Medicine*, 7, 1-15

Wellisch, P.K., Jamison, K.R. and Pasnau, R.O. (1978) 'Psychosocial Aspects of Mastectomy, II: The man's perspective', *American Journal of Psychiatry*, 135, 543-6

Wilbur, G.M. (1983) 'Mastectomy Nursing', *Nursing Times*, 29 June, 66-7

Wilkinson, S., Maguire, P., Tait, A., Brooke, M., Faulkner, A. and Sellwood, R. (1983) 'A Comparison of Three Methods of Counselling and Monitoring Women who Undergo Mastectomy', Proceedings of International Conference: *Research — A Base For The Future?*, University of Edinburgh, Nursing Studies Research Unit

Wing, J.K. Cooper, J.E. and Sartorious, N. (1974) *Measurement and Classification of Psychiatric Symptoms*, Cambridge University Press: Cambridge

Winnick, L. and Robbins, G. (1977) 'Physical and Psychological Adjustment After Mastectomy', *Cancer*, 39, 478

Witkin, M.H. (1978) 'Psychosexual Counselling of the Mastectomy Patient', *Journal of Sex and Marital Therapy*, 4, 20-8

Woods, N.F. and Earp, J.A. (1978) 'Women with Cured Breast Cancer', *Nursing Research*, 27, 279-85

Worden, L.W. and Weisman, A.D. (1977) 'The Fallacy of Post-mastectomy Depression', *The American Journal of the Medical Sciences*, 273, 169-75

Yasko, J.M. (1983) 'Variables which Predict Burnout Experienced by Oncology Clinical Nurse Specialists', *Cancer Nursing*, 6, 109-16

PART V:

TEACHING INTERPERSONAL SKILLS TO NURSES

EDITORIAL INTRODUCTION

One of the most persistent themes to emerge from the previous sections, is the need for training in interpersonal skills. Indeed, different authors have suggested different methods of doing this.

Experiential methods give learners the opportunity to engage actively in their learning, and *Anne Tomlinson* considers the relative merits of a variety of teaching methods in *Chapter 12*. As she points out, verbal and non-verbal skills are a part of everyday life: the professional skill is to know when and why to use particular strategies and how to manage the effects they have. The insight, personal awareness and appreciation of group relationships that can derive from experiential learning should help nurses develop these professional skills. Just as there are psychological, physical and organisational barriers to the effective use of interpersonal skills, so there are barriers to effective interpersonal skill learning: a plea is made for nurse educators at all levels to take these into account. The role of the teacher using experiential methods is of facilitator rather than instructor (although, as Tomlinson points out, there is room for some didactic components of a teaching package) and this, in itself, requires particular teaching skills. Both teachers and learners may have emotional experiences in the classroom, and it is the teachers' responsibility to deal with this constructively at the time. Coping with crisis in the classroom is something that nurse teachers may not have met before, and it is as well to be prepared in advance. Tomlinson also stresses the importance of good relationships with colleagues, especially those in clinical areas, so that the school-taught skills may be practised in clinical settings. Ultimately the choice of teaching method will depend on the subject matter being taught — different topics lend themselves to different methods, and different groups of students will respond more readily to different styles of learning.

This point is pursued by the following three authors, who discuss their experiences of teaching interpersonal skills to nurses undertaking different forms of training.

In *Chapter 13, Gary Marshfield* presents some thoughts on introducing interpersonal skills into general nurse training. Before incorporating interpersonal skills sessions, Marshfield urges that five

)

central questions should be considered: what should be *taught*? What kind of *content*? How much *time* is available? How should sessions be structured? and what *methods* should be used? He favours a mixture of experiential learning and structured handout material. In order to stimulate group discussion, he makes extensive use of 'trigger materials': as long as the group size is no more than 14 he finds this encourages full participation. For students to be able to engage in their (often noisy) work, the entire learning context must be examined, and suitable premises obtained. Marshfield presents a summary of his course as it has developed and gives some examples of student reactions to it in terms of their own personal growth. He goes on to discuss the implications of interpersonal skills teaching for teachers, and draws attention to the ethical issues that are involved, the resources that are necessary and the training needs of teachers. Finally he notes the importance of formal and informal support systems for both teachers and students.

The implications of interpersonal skills teaching for nurse teachers are highlighted, too, by *Bill Reynolds (Chapter 14)* in the context of psychiatric nurse training. He takes as his starting point the need to discard the 'medical model' of nursing in favour of a counselling model. One consequence of this is that teachers must be prepared to take risks with students and develop their own levels of self-awareness. They will then be able to create a non-threatening learning context that will facilitate students' personal growth. If the attitudinal and behavioural changes sought by teachers in their students are to occur, Reynolds urges that teachers practise what they preach: one way for them to do this would be for them to hold joint teaching clinical posts. Reynolds suggests several teaching tools that can usefully be used, in conjunction with experiential methods, to structure and induce learning.

Whilst Reynolds adopts a counselling model, and discusses the development of counselling skills, in *Chapter 15, Carolyn Kagan* employs an eclectic model of social interaction to plan various interpersonal skills courses for nurses as part of their post-basic training. The students on these courses all have different needs, varying experiences of nursing and are usually following tightly-packed syllabi leading to formal assessment. Kagan shares her experiences of teaching students who differ in a number of ways in their approaches to interpersonal skills learning: those who are highly motivated and those who are not; those who see interpersonal skills as a legitimate part of their work and training and those who do not; those who are able to devote a considerable amount of time to interpersonal skills learning and those who are not; and those who require a substantial theoretical input to their course and those who do not. She points out that the professional validating bodies differ in the extent to which they identify specific interpersonal skills that students should be expected to have acquired, on completion of their course. Furthermore, the relative importance they attribute to interpersonal skills components, within the overall course syllabi and assessments, in part determines student attitudes towards the learning. Kagan also discusses issues arising out of organisational structures, such as class size, assessment requirements and tutor limitations.

Ann Faulkner develops the theme of assessment and evaluation in *Chapter 16*. She draws a distinction between attempts to discover whether underlying concepts have been understood — which can be through written material — and attempts to assess whether the skills have been learnt — which can be through the analysis of audio, audio-visual or actual interactions. Methodological rigour will require that such interaction analysis will be reliable, and this will have implications for the training of raters. Ideally, experimental studies of teaching/ learning will include before- and after-teaching measures of skill, pre- ferably with some follow-up assessment. Thus the resource implications of the experimental evaluation of teaching/learning are considerable. Other, less stringent possibilities for evaluation, including patient assessment, are discussed. Whichever system of evaluation is used, the outcome measures must be clearly specified, and realistic with regard to the specific teaching objectives. In the end, though, interpersonal skills teaching (and learning) will depend on the quality of that teaching, and Faulkner has established the training of teachers to be a priority.

12 THE USE OF EXPERIENTIAL METHODS IN TEACHING INTERPERSONAL SKILLS TO NURSES

Anne Tomlinson

Introduction

During twenty-six years of working within the National Health Service I have observed, experienced and, I fear, practised ineffective communication. The course of study leading to the Diploma in Nursing introduced me to a wealth of research demonstrating problems of communication within the health service. I read of poor interpersonal communication (Altschul, 1972; Stockwell, 1972); ineffective group communication (Lelean, 1973); patient dissatisfaction with communication (Cartwright, 1964) and later, increased satisfaction with care and improved patient recovery where communication is encouraged (Boore, 1978; Hayward, 1975; Wilson-Barnett, 1978). I also observed that in spite of research findings, further studies continued to demonstrate that communication between health care professionals and their patients needed improvement (Ashworth, 1980; Cormack, 1976; Macleod Clark, 1981).

On entering the field of Nurse Education, I became aware of the difficulties and problems inherent in attempts to teach interpersonal communication to nursing students. I found an even greater challenge when confronted with evaluating a nurse's ability to communicate with others. During my experience in nurse education I have heard and used anecdotes and clichés in an attempt to encourage students to demonstrate a humanistic approach to patients. Phrases such as 'treat your patients like guests', 'listen to your patients', 'make your patient comfortable', 'reassure your patient', and 'try to meet your patient's psychological needs', have reverberated around schools of nursing from the lips of myself and others. It soon became clear to me that if I wanted to influence nurses' attitudes or help them develop their interpersonal skills, I needed to explore more appropriate methods to achieve these aims. This search led me toward 'experiential methods', a wide range of teaching methods which involve the student in a high degree of active participation in the learning process. McFarlane

191

(1976) advocated the use of methods which offer the student 'feeling experiences', Williams (1978) wrote about the value of role-play, and French (1980) suggested the use of simulation to provide students with meaningful learning experiences. These and other methods which encourage interaction between individual students and teachers, and provide opportunities to explore actions and the feelings generated by them, are becoming increasingly accepted in nurse education as valuable tools for achieving personal growth and attitude change.

I found that students enjoyed this type of learning and said that they learned a great deal from 'feeling what it is like to be a patient'. I also found that through small-group work and classroom interaction, students said that their confidence increased and their creativity was encouraged. Through classroom discussion their self-awareness grew and attitudes appeared to change. Sadly I did not attempt to evaluate this learning formally. Since then I have learned a great deal, some of which I intend to share in this chapter.

At present I am involved with a research project (CINE, funded by the Health Education Council), which is attempting to teach communication skills to student nurses, and to evaluate the effectiveness of the teaching by measuring changes in student knowledge, attitudes and SKILLS in communicating as health care professionals. It is from this background and experience that I find the motivation to contribute this chapter.

Professional Communication

According to Mackenzie (1971, p.42), one of the hallmarks of a profession is

> ... an occupation whose activities are subject to constant critical analysis — so far as the purpose of the occupation is concerned. A profession in fact is never static; there is continuous change and development and a discarding of what is of less use in favour of what is more use.

The adoption of the nursing process, with its systematic approach including problem-solving and evaluation of care, has caused many nurses to question the effectiveness of professional communication in nursing. The research studies cited above have demonstrated the ineffectiveness of much professional communication, and recommendations for changes leading to improvement have been made. Professional communication in nursing differs from everyday communication in a number of ways, including the problem-solving nature of the encounter; the role differences of the participants and their preconceived expectations; the clinical environment and potential seriousness of the meeting (for the patient); the mental or physical discomfort of the patient and the professional responsibility of the nurse to instigate action to relieve it. It is essential, therefore, that a nurse obtains and gives accurate information in order to achieve effective professional communication.

Nurses need to be able to use a systematic approach in order to work with their patient to identify problems, plan nursing care, implement actions and evaluate their effectiveness. To enable them to do this nurses also need an understanding of the nature of nursing and the nurse's professional role. If the nursing process is an activity which centres around the patient, and accepts his/her individual freedom to become involved in his/her care and make decisions related to that care, nurses, then, require an understanding of what is meant by patient-centred activities. This in turn requires a knowledge of human behaviour which includes self-awareness, an awareness of others, awareness of group processes and how an individual's knowledge, skills and attitudes can affect human interactions. The nursing process is founded on the concept of a 'caring', 'helping', interpersonal relationship, in which the nurses should be able to separate their own needs from those of their patients in order to concentrate their attention on meeting the patients' needs.

Barriers to Effective Communication

Communication requires two people, each a unique individual, from different backgrounds, who may be of different sex, age, culture and social class. Each person receives information through five physiological senses and interprets messages through physical and psychological processes. The passage of information is a continuous process between the two participants, the information being interpreted by each individual based on assumptions evolved from a multitude of past experiences and interactions. Even in the absence of physical or psychological disability there can be many barriers or disruptions to effective communication. The use of 'blocking tactics', unclear messages, contradictory non-verbal behaviour, inaccurate feedback and insensitivity are just some of the many examples available. Where physical or psychological disability, prejudice, disruptive environmental factors such as noise, heat, cold and unmet basic needs exist, then the barriers to effective communication will be even greater. This is illustrated in Figure 12.1. If nurses are distracted by their own physical or psychological needs, or if their ability to communicate is blocked by defence mechanisms outlined by Menzies (1960), they will be unable to offer their patients the interpersonal relationship the nursing process demands.

It is becoming increasingly apparent from the results of research findings that a greater proportion of time and attention, assigned to meeting students' educational needs, should be devoted to this aspect of nurse education.

Communication Skills

For convenience, human communication behaviour can be divided into two categories, those which involve verbal skills, and those which involve non-verbal skills. There is considerable variation in the way specific skills are identified, which seems to be related to the training approach being used. For the purpose of this chapter I have identified them under the following categories:

Linguistic and paralinguistic skills, which include
    the clear and precise use of language
    tone of voice
    pitch, inflection, volume and speed of speech
Non-verbal skills, which include the use of

eye contact	body orientation
touch	personal space or distance
facial expression	speed of movement
gesture	general appearance
body posture	

Skills which involve elements from both of these categories plus the intent with which they are used, and which include

listening	eliciting information
attending	giving information
responding	comforting
encouraging	reassuring

The intentional way language is used can have more or less helpful outcomes:

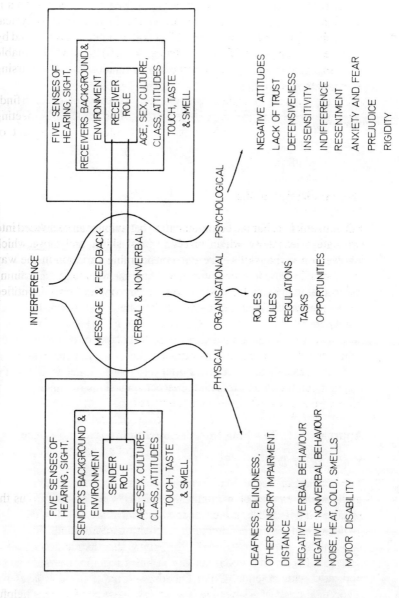

BARRIERS TO EFFECTIVE COMMUNICATION

FIVE SENSES OF HEARING, SIGHT.

RECEIVER'S BACKGROUND & ENVIRONMENT

RECEIVER ROLE

AGE, SEX, CULTURE, CLASS, ATTITUDES

TOUCH, TASTE & SMELL

INTERFERENCE

MESSAGE & FEEDBACK

VERBAL & NONVERBAL

FIVE SENSES OF HEARING, SIGHT.

SENDER'S BACKGROUND & ENVIRONMENT

SENDER ROLE

AGE, SEX, CULTURE, CLASS, ATTITUDES

TOUCH, TASTE & SMELL

PHYSICAL

DEAFNESS. BLINDNESS.
OTHER SENSORY IMPAIRMENT
DISTANCE
NEGATIVE VERBAL BEHAVIOUR
NEGATIVE NONVERBAL BEHAVIOUR
NOISE, HEAT, COLD, SMELLS
MOTOR DISABILITY

ORGANISATIONAL

ROLES
RULES
REGULATIONS
TASKS
OPPORTUNITIES

PSYCHOLOGICAL

NEGATIVE ATTITUDES
LACK OF TRUST
DEFENSIVENESS
INSENSITIVITY
INDIFFERENCE
RESENTMENT
ANXIETY AND FEAR
PREJUDICE
RIGIDITY

Helpful	*Unhelpful*
praising	blaming
accepting	distracting
clarifying	ignoring
demonstrating interest	evading
offering support	rejecting
avoiding euphemisms	demanding
avoiding ambiguities	using jargon

Some strategies we use can fall into both of these categories, for example,

criticising
challenging
agreeing
apologising
voicing doubt

The use of verbal and non-verbal skills, tactics and strategies of behaviour is part and parcel of everyday life. The skill comes from being aware of when and why we are using these strategies and knowing how to manage the outcomes resulting from their use. Nursing research has shown that many nurses use strategies which block communication between themselves and the people they care for (Ashworth, 1980; Faulkner, 1981; Hawker, 1982; Macleod Clark, 1981). There is a need for nurses to become aware of the skilful use of communication behaviour, the blocks that can occur, and how they may be overcome. Different theoretical approaches offer different techniques and methods that can be used in teaching interpersonal skills to nurses.

Approaches to Teaching Interpersonal Skills

Social Skills Training (SST)

The concept of Social Skill Training centres around the notion that social skills consist of a number of subskills which can be easily acquired. These subskills have become known as micro-skills, which, if identified and practised individually can be combined and incorporated into skilled behaviour. Argyle (1981) states that, like a motor skill, a social skill is an intentional activity, it has a specific aim and can be improved with practice. Colin Davidson (Chapter 2) discusses the theoretical basis of SST.

Teachers working within this framework plan skill training which includes the identification of individual micro-skills, observation or demonstration of skilled performance, practice of the skill by the learners and feedback to the learners regarding their degree of success. This process is repeated until the trainer and trainee are satisfied with the outcome. The bulk of research into SST has been in the psychiatric field (e.g. Spence and Shepherd, 1983), but it has also been used extensively in three other areas of need; remedial training with handicapped people, developmental training during educational courses, and specialised training for professional development (Ellis and Whittington, 1981).

It is only recently that nurse educators have recognised the value of identifying micro-skills and including SST in educational courses.

Analytic Approaches

Sigmund Freud proposed a theory of personality development and behaviour based on the assumption that human behaviour stems from unconscious processes. This theory suggested that impulses, derived from innate instincts, are driven into the unconscious through being forbidden by society or punished by parents during a child's socialisation. These repressed unconscious impulses, Freud suggests, can be expressed through slips of speech, in dreams, and in mannerisms. They can also be channelled unconsciously into artistic activities or remain repressed to affect behaviour. This basic idea has led to the development of several methods of treating mental illness, based on the process of Psychoanalysis, and has also formed the basis of an explanation of human interactions, namely Transactional Analysis (Berne, 1976). Berne, using the concept of 'Ego States' from Freud's theory, analysed human interactions in terms of Child, Parent and Adult behaviour. Other concepts within Berne's theory include 'Life Positions', 'Scripts', 'Games', 'Strokes', 'Rackets', and 'Drivers'. Each of these concepts offers explanations of interpersonal behaviour and can be used for helping students increase their awareness of interactive processes. Levin (1972) contributed to an understanding of nursing behaviour in her article 'Games Nurses Play'. Transactional Analysis, while a complex theory, offers nursing a framework for analysing nursing behaviour. It can be used in the classroom with groups in conjunction with videotaped nurse-patient interactions, transcripts of nurse-patient conversations and role-play.

Humanistic Approaches

The third theoretical perspective that offers useful teaching methods for nurse educators is the humanistic or phenomenological approach. This perspective focuses on the individual's own perception and interpretation of events — his/her subjective experience. It encompasses the notion that people should be studied through their own individual experience, without the application of theoretical ideas or psychological preconceptions. The humanistic approach is concerned with self direction and freedom of choice, it emphasises the positive aspect of people and their individual drives toward self-actualisation. It is within this approach to psychology that Carl Rogers and others have developed the activity known as non-directive counselling. This approach to counselling is based on the assumption that the unique individual can, with help, identify his or her problems and make decisions regarding positive change.

Methods offered by humanistic psychology are based on the premise that there is a need to encourage self-awareness, and that through self-awareness an understanding of others will develop. This can be achieved through training ('T') groups, individual counselling, experiential exercises, simulations and role-play. Personal life experiences can be explored using what is known as the 'critical incident' technique, and another technique known as 'sculpting'.

Ways of Teaching Interpersonal Skills

There are a wide variety of methods available for use in the teaching of interpersonal skills, and they include:

Lectures

All learning requires a knowledge base from which a student can build an understanding of complex processes. Didactic teaching can be effective in encouraging cognitive learning, passing on theoretical principles and making essential introductions to a topic. Students arrive for training with widely varying levels of knowledge, and many teachers feel that by providing an introductory lecture they ensure that all students have the same knowledge base from which to begin further exploration of a subject. This assumption fails to take account of the fact that people differ in the ways they acquire knowledge and that, for some, lectures may be ineffective. While lectures may be appropriate for more academically motivated students, many others can be helped to achieve the same knowledge level using more interactive methods.

Discussions

Many students who have poor concentration, or those who respond to active involvement with others, frequently state a preference for discussion-based learning. Argyle (1973) suggests that discussion can play a useful part in teaching social skill. He does, however, say that discussion is better combined with demonstrations, exercises, films, role-playing and experiments. For me, the less formal atmosphere created by group discussion is more appropriate to the humanistic approach I prefer to adopt. If teachers are attempting to encourage a humanistic nurse-patient relationship, a similar teacher-student relationship should be demonstrated in the classroom. King and Gerwig (1981) outline how a humanistic approach to nurse education can be achieved through group process.

Role-Play

Role-play has been shown to be one of the most effective methods of training in social skills, particularly in the areas of Industrial Relations and Management (Argyle, 1973). In nurse education, French (1980) encourages the use of role-play for enabling learners to experience their own feelings in emergency or emotionally difficult situations. Farrell, Haley and Magnasco (1977) showed that, following a planned course using intensive role-play exercises, students in the experimental group 'increased their facilitative interpersonal ability', when measured on a Carkhuff rating scale. The use of role-play as a learning experience has become a valuable tool in the education of health care professionals (Ellis and Whittington, 1981). At an interpersonal level, role-play can be used to identify personal behaviour patterns and try out new behaviours before accepting change. Role-play can provide opportunities for students to experience what it may be like to be a patient subjected to specific procedures, e.g. admission to hospital, bed bathing, isolation or preparation for surgery. It could include simulating blindness, physical handicap and confinement to a wheelchair (Williams, 1978). Role-play aims to provide the learner with those 'feeling experiences' advocated by McFarlane (1976), and leads the learner to understand the situation of others, their roles, relationships and attitudes (French, 1980).

Role-play has also been shown to allow students to experience the pressures which create roles, and to recognise how roles are both adopted by the individual and imposed on a person by others (van Ments, 1978); to facilitate the development of self-awareness and heighten sensitivity (van Ments, 1978); and to motivate learners to examine their own behaviour and, where appropriate, effect change (Rackham and Morgan, 1971). Role-play can improve teaching skills and heighten recognition of the need to use lay language in patient education (King and Gerwig, 1981), and it provides opportunities for practising the skills and behaviours appropriate to other roles (Sundeen, Stuart, Rankin and Cohen, 1981). Clark (1978) suggests that role-playing helps students understand the behaviour of, and develop tolerance toward, others, as well as releasing emotional tension through the expression of personal opinions and exploration of individuals' feelings. At the group level, role-play can demonstrate, more clearly than words, lines of communication and power structures; it can pave the way to the development of warm open relationships within the group leading to group unity and the production of effective working relationships. Finally it helps to bridge the gap between cognitive learning and affective behaviour.

Simulations and Games

Most simulations and games are structured to include goals, resources, constraints, activities and pay-offs (Clark, 1978). They can be individual or group activities. They are commonly used to give learners experience of job interviews, disciplinary procedures, dismissals, management and emergency situations. They give students insight into the effect of negative and positive attitudes, and can lead to increased competence in specific situations. Simulations can be used to encourage the development of problem-solving skills and the use of creativity, and have been used extensively in assertiveness training (Trower, Bryant and Argyle, 1978). Specific simulations frequently include the use of role-play by the participants.

Critical Incident Technique

Outlined by Flanagan (1954), this technique draws on the personal experiences of individual members of a group. Students are asked to recall a situation they have experienced which has caused them pleasure, anxiety, annoyance or other emotional effects. This method can be particularly useful in exploring the clinical experiences of learners. These can be used in several ways. If every member is asked to contribute an experience, they can be written down briefly, mixed to provide anonymity, and read by another member of the group. Alternatively, experiences can be handed to the group leader to select one or two. Contributions can be discussed, or role-played, with group members offering thoughts, feelings or alternative ways of responding to the situation.

Sculpting

This is another way of using learners' individual experiences. It is a way of encouraging non-verbal, physical demonstration of an interactional situation. One member of the group volunteers to contribute a personal experience, visualising the attitudes and positions of those involved. Other group members are then chosen to recreate the positions and attitudes of the people described by the contributor. The members posing as 'statues' in the scene are asked to try to imagine how it feels to be the person they are depicting. When the sculpt is complete, time is allowed for the group to take in and imagine the real situation which produced it. The sculpt is then discussed, with the participants contributing their feelings and impressions to the group. The group leader encourages members to offer alternative behaviours which could have been used to provide positive outcomes. Houston (1979) found the use of sculpts valuable to demonstrate relationships within a group, and suggested it is a way of making a fantasy real. An alternative way of using sculpts is to encourage group members all to take part in the sculpt, negotiating with each other their positions and relationships within the group. Sculpting can prove a powerful tool that may generate strong emotional experiences for those involved.

Training Groups

Training, or 'T' groups centre on the concepts of sensitivity and awareness. They take a variety of forms and include descriptions such as 'sensitivity training', 'encounter group', 'Tavistock Group' (as promoted by the Tavistock Institute), and 'process group'. Training groups can serve a variety of functions. Some aim to bring about an increase in awareness of personal functioning; they can help individuals become more aware of the feelings and attitudes of others, and they may lead to an increase in self acceptance and understanding. Some aim to encourage members to explore group interactions and facilitate the development of alternative behaviours in difficult life or work situations. Argyle (1973), gives a comprehensive assessment of T-group training: many studies are quoted and wide variations in the effectiveness of this approach have been found. While some group members have been reported to benefit from group training, others have developed serious problems. Underwood (1965) found that one trainee became less effective for every two who became more effective. Results of studies into T-group training have been inconclusive but suggest that members high in anxiety and defensiveness are most likely to become emotionally disturbed. Argyle and Kendon (1967) note that adolescents are particularly insecure, as they are unsure of their self image. If this is so it may be more appropriate to offer T-group training as an alternative optional addition to general nurse training, or leave it until later in the course when students have become familiar with, and competent at, basic nursing procedures. It may also be necessary to be selective when making decisions about who attends T-group training, with only those who are likely to benefit most being encouraged to attend. If learning experiences risk emotional trauma for the participants, strong support systems are necessary for the trainees. Unless tutors in schools for general nurse training can offer this support, or have the skills which encourage students to support each other when experiencing stress, caution regarding T-group work should be exercised. Many of the successful outcomes resulting from T-group training can be achieved using methods already described.

Summary of Approaches

It is widely accepted in education that individual learning is increased when the student is actively involved in the learning process. Experiential methods are those which involve the student in a high degree of active participation in the learning activity. They encourage interaction between individual students and tutor, and they also encourage those involved to examine both their feelings and behaviour. As entrants to nurse training have already been experiencing communication for many years, it is necessary to convince them that professional communication differs from everyday communication in a number of ways. Owing to the fact that all students have a multitude of life experiences on which to draw, it is likely that cognitive learning can be achieved without the need for formal lectures. Individualised learning, including reading references, handouts, structured exercises, small-group work and brainstorming within a discussion group setting, should provide the knowledge base necessary.

The choice of teaching method will depend on the style of the teachers, their awareness of their own skills, students' learning needs and preferences, and the appropriateness of the method for achieving the aims of the course or session. Many of the studies referenced are from work in social psychology, industrial relations and management training. There is a great need for research into the effectiveness of specific teaching methods in achieving the aims of sessions or courses in nurse education. Due to the ages of nursing students, and other pressures on them during training, methods appropriate for other courses may not prove so effective when used for student nurses. There is also a need to be aware that the democratic styles of behaviour frequently taught during courses based on a solely humanistic approach may be inappropriate when learners return to a hierarchical and authoritarian organisation.

Optimising the Success of Experiential Learning

The Classroom Environment

If nurse educators are hoping to encourage effective communication between nurses and patients or colleagues, the teacher is compelled to look at the relationship between teacher and student. There is considerable similarity between the teacher-student relationship and the nurse-patient relationship. In each case, one is assisting the other to meet individual needs, to identify problems and provide solutions. In both cases there is a need to develop help-seeking, help-accepting and problem-solving behaviours. It is therefore necessary for the teacher to provide a more comfortable and humanistic classroom atmosphere than many tutors and students have experienced in the past.

The decision to use experiential methods in interpersonal skills teaching has implications for both the teacher and learners. When learners are physically or psychologically uncomfortable the learning process may be inhibited; it is the responsibility of the teacher to provide a comfortable learning environment. This can prove difficult when teachers are faced with meeting a wide variety of student needs. Physical comfort can be achieved through thoughtful planning: sessions should include changes in activity, breaks, and comfortable seating, especially if the session is discussion based. Room temperature and lighting can be negotiated to meet majority needs. Visual aids such as trigger tapes, handouts, slides and incident cards, all help to maintain motivation in the students.

Psychological comfort presents a greater challenge. All students enter nursing at a different stage in their cognitive, affective and skills development. Some students have high academic qualifications, others do not; some are outgoing, others reserved; some students demonstrate highly developed interpersonal skills, others less. To enable students to speak freely within a group environment it is necessary for teachers to be aware of their own psychological comfort, which can act to increase or inhibit their communication skills with students. Teachers, whether they are aware of it or not, act as models for students. King and Gerwig (1981, p.100) state,

> Although experiential learning through the use of diad and triad role-playing is valuable, the most effective way in which a teacher can teach understanding, respect, warmth, and genuineness is to demonstrate these qualities herself.

Teachers need to be skilled observers of the whole group, and sensitive to the feelings of individual students. They should be aware of the dynamics of the group and able to use group processes as learning experiences for students. Sensitive responses to students' experiences help to provide a comfortable psychological environment in the classroom.

Reducing Emotional Arousal

Learning reaches a peak at a specific point of emotional arousal. If the level of emotional arousal caused by the psychological environment in the classroom is too high, student learning may be reduced. On the other hand there must be sufficient emotional stimulation to motivate learners to achieve optimum learning. As the needs of individual students vary widely, it is probable that the teacher will be unable to meet them all. This may, inevitably, lead to difficulties for some students. Where this occurs the perceptive teacher will recognise students' problems and take action to enable these individuals to overcome them. Western culture has a tendency to discourage people from being open about their attitudes and feelings. By the time people arrive for nurse training they have been through a process of socialisation which has, for some, encouraged the formation of elaborate defence mechanisms. A student who has a 'reserved' personality may find it difficult to speak in front of a group. A student who has grown up subjected to criticism may have a weak self image and be defensive when receiving feedback from the group. The teacher can do much to increase the self image of individual students through the use of praise, approval and encouragement. This is important when the teacher recognises that a particularly reticent student is taking a personal risk by making a contribution to the session.

It is important for students to be given time and attention when attempting to put into words ideas they are having difficulty expressing.

Teachers themselves, and other students, may well discourage a reluctant student by 'jumping in' and filling any small silences there may be during a session. It is necessary for the teacher to take steps to control more vocal members and demonstrate the use of positive feedback to students. Actions taken should not cause a student to feel 'put down' and quiet students can be encouraged by being invited to participate. This can sometimes cause a sensitive student to feel the focus of attention, and result in embarrassment, but if the teacher can generate a light-hearted atmosphere, this can have very positive outcomes for the group.

Development of Self-Awareness

Experiential methods are frequently used to encourage students to explore their feelings. The use of these methods can also expose behaviours and attitudes which the learner may wish to remain unseen. As there is personal danger to both the student and teacher when this occurs, either may find it difficult to make disclosures of a private nature. Allowing others to see things about us which are normally hidden, involves an element of risk. These risks are more likely to be taken in a relatively safe environment and are frequently related to loss of face, loss of control and loss of friendship. It is the responsibility of the teacher to minimise these risks. If group members who take risks and demonstrate a negative aspect of behaviour are criticised, they will experience loss of face in front of their peers. However, if they are helped to feel that the particular behaviour is common to both the teacher and other group members the learner will feel supported. Encouraging supporting strategies from group members also helps to form close relationships within the group. Sometimes students undertaking a specific role-play touch on a subject which has particular emotional meaning for a particular student. It could be something experienced in private life or during a clinical experience. This may cause an emotional reaction from the student leading to loss of control, either tears or a display of anger. As before, if the group is encouraged to support this student then the risk to him/her is reduced. In these situations students should be encouraged to discuss the event and the emotions which caused it but only if they feel that it is comfortable to do so. For many individuals there are some things which must remain confidential, and students should be enabled to feel free to withold whatever they wish. If a session has included a particularly emotional or difficult experience, it can be useful to end the session with each member of the group taking a turn at telling each other member something they like about him/her. This concludes the session on a positive note and helps to maintain the friendly relationships which existed before the session.

Self-awareness can also be increased through introspection which involves questioning one's own attitudes, motivations and feelings. The use of experiential methods can encourage a speeding-up of the process, through the shared experiences of the simulated situation. It will be more painful for the learner, the more public the setting in which the learning occurs. Students may need some theoretical knowledge of the importance of self-awareness to enable them to recognise the value of experiential classroom learning. Egan (1977) offers useful material for students as background reading.

Relating Classroom Activities to Ward Experience

Exercises which students can undertake in clinical areas bridge the gap between theory and practice. It is helpful to give students time to observe ward activities and interactions without being part of the ward team. This helps them to identify barriers to communication in the clinical area, and enables them to think through the problems and provide possible solutions. Group discussion of ward observation helps students to recognise differences and similarities between wards and the interpersonal relationships which occur throughout the hierarchy. Exercises can be designed that encourage students to practise specific skills. Those which focus on 'listening', 'attending and responding', 'questioning', 'encouraging', 'giving information', 'opening, controlling and closing conversations', and offering 'comfort and reassurance', are particularly useful. Each skill can be practised in the classroom using role-play with students working in two's and three's practising, observing and assessing each other's level of skill. The same exercise can then be tried in the clinical area with patients filling the 'patient roles'. In each case a tape recorder can be used to capture the simulated exercise. Recordings are extremely useful as they provide a transcript of the conversation which makes feedback and analysis more accurate. They also provide a record of skill development for individual students which can help to increase their confidence. Other methods of process recording are discussed by Bill Reynolds (Chapter 14). Students frequently comment that both role-play and ward-based exercises seem artificial. It is necessary to stress the value of practice in the development of interpersonal skill. All feedback to students should concentrate on the positive aspects of performance, and self assessment should be encouraged. Feedback must be handled with sensitivity and where a student is particularly vulnerable it should be given in a private setting. It is useful to encourage students to share their experiences in these practice settings: sensitively managed group discussion can help the more negative student recognise the value of skills practice.

The use of clinical areas for practice exercises depends on good working relationships between teachers and other members of the care team. If the use of tape recorders is planned, it may be necessary to obtain permission of medical, nursing administration and ward staff, as well as patients. All recorded material must be treated as highly confidential and the anonymity of patients preserved.

Coping with Crisis

Internal group dynamics, and events within the programme of training but outside the control of the interpersonal skills teacher, can have a profound effect on the responses of students within a session using experiential methods. Friction between individuals in a group can raise issues which require attention within the classroom setting. Anger generated by occurrences outside the classroom is sometimes brought to the attention of the interpersonal skills teacher. It is vital that these issues are given the time and attention of the teacher, otherwise students' problems will be left unresolved and skills sessions may be seriously disrupted. Attention to these difficulties necessitates a considerable degree of openness on the part of the teacher, who must be prepared to explore any issue that students raise. This involves skilful classroom management, as the teacher must also recognise when students are using tactics to divert attention away from the objectives of the session. Physical games which allow students to make a noise and use up aggressive energy can be helpful in dissipating tensions. The teacher should be able to use conflict and confrontation in a positive way to help students recognise the function of these concepts in interpersonal relationships.

Conclusion

Interpersonal relationships and professional communication are a much overlooked area of nursing education. It is necessary to develop a curriculum which pays much greater attention to these issues, and experiential methods, involving the students actively in the learning experience, are the most appropriate methods to use when teaching about human relationships.

There are many 'key concepts' which should be covered during any course on human relationships; a list of these appears at the end of this chapter. Barriers to communication should be identified and ways of overcoming them explained. Interpersonal communication consists of a number of skills which can be placed into verbal, non-verbal and general categories. Students need to be aware that skills are intentional acts which can be developed with practice and that highly developed skills improve interpersonal relationships.

There are a wide range of experiential methods suitable for use in interpersonal skills teaching. The selection of a particular method will depend on whether specific skills development, increased self-awareness or more general learning is envisaged. A combination of methods is probably the most effective way of meeting the needs of a wide variety of students. The provision of an atmosphere of psychological safety is one of the most challenging aspects of this type of teaching. It is possible to achieve this through skilful classroom management, personal comfort with the teaching methods used, and a willingness to develop interpersonal relationships with the students being taught.

It is important for students to understand the relationship between learning in the classroom and clinical experience. Teachers can bridge this gap by providing students with ward-based learning exercises but this requires cooperation from other members of the health care team, and tests the relationship-building skill of the teacher.

Because sessions which encourage students to examine interpersonal relationships encourage the expression of feelings, high levels of emotion may be experienced. The teacher must have the skill and confidence to deal with emotionally charged situations and provide students with a comfortable working environment in which any issue raised can be explored. This may mean that the interpersonal skills teachers should take part in some training sessions themselves and experience experiential learning at first hand. As a general rule, they should not ask students to do anything that they have not done and would not be prepared to do themselves. The management of interpersonal skills teaching is one of the most challenging issues facing nurse educators today.

Key Concepts Worthy of Examination in any Interpersonal Skills Teaching Programme:

ACCOUNTABILITY	DEFENCE	POWER
ADVOCACY	DENIAL	PRAISE
ANGER	DEPENDENCE	PROBLEM-SOLVING
ANXIETY	DETACHMENT	
ASSERTIVENESS	DIAGNOSIS	QUESTIONING
ASSESSMENT		
ATTENTION	EDUCATION	
ATTENDING	EMPATHY	REASSURANCE
ATTITUDES	ENCOURAGEMENT	REJECTION
AUTHORITY		RELATIONSHIP
	FRUSTRATION	RESPONDING
		RIGHTS
BARRIERS	HEALTH	ROLES
BEHAVIOUR	HIERARCHY	
		SELF
CLARIFICATION	LISTENING	SELF-AWARENESS
CLASS		SHARING
COMFORT	NEEDS	SKILLS — verbal
COMMUNICATION	NURSE	non-verbal
CONFIDENCE	NURSE CENTRED	STATUS
CONFLICT		
CONFRONTATION	ORGANISATION	TEACHER
CONTROL		TRUST
CUES — verbal	PATIENT	
non-verbal	PATIENT CENTRED	
CULTURE	PATRONISING	VALUING

References

Altschul, A. (1972) *Patient-Nurse Interaction*, Churchill Livingston: Edinburgh

Argyle, M. (ed.) (1981) *Social Skills and Health*, Methuen; London

Argyle, M. (1973) *Social Interaction*, Tavistock Publications: London

Argyle, M. and Kendon, A. (1967) 'The Experimental Analysis of Social Performance', in L. Berkowitz (ed.) *Advances in Experimental Social Psychology, 3*, Academic Press: New York

Ashworth, P. (1980) *Care to Communicate*, RCN: London

Berne, E. (1976) *Games People Play*, Penguin: Harmondsworth

Boore, J. (1978) *A Prescription for Recovery*, RCN: London

Cartwright, A. (1964) *Human Relations and Hospital Care*, Routledge and Kegan Paul: London

Cormack, D. (1976) *Psychiatric Nursing Observed*, RCN: London

Clark, C.C. (1978) *Classroom Skills for Nurse Educators*, Springer: New York

Egan, G. (1977) *You & Me*, Brooks/Cole: California

Ellis, R. and Whittington, D. (1981) *A Guide to Social Skill Training*, Croom Helm: London

Farrell, M., Haley, M. and Magnasco, J. (1977) 'Teaching Interpersonal Skills', *Nursing Outlook, 25*, 322-5

Faulkner, A. (1981) 'Aye, There's the Rub', *Nursing Times, 77*, 332-6

Flanagan, J.C. (1954) 'The Critical Incident Technique', *Psychological Bulletin, 51*, 327-58

French, H.P. (1980) 'A Place for Simulation in Nurse Education', *Nursing Focus*, July, 445-6

Hawker, R. (1982) *Interaction Between Nurses and Patients' Relatives*, Paper at RCN Research Conference, Durham

Hayward, J. (1975) *Information, A Prescription Against Pain*, RCN: London

Houston, G. (1979) *All in the Mind*: The making of an interpersonal group in a television series, BBC Publications: London

King, V.G. and Gerwig, N.A. (1981) *Humanising Nursing Education: A confluent approach through group process*, Nursing Resources: Wakefield Mass.

Lelean, S. (1973) *Ready for Report Nurse?*, RCN: London

Levin, P. (1972) 'Games Nurses Play', *American Journal of Nursing, 72*, 483-7

Mackenzie, N. (1971) *The Professional Ethic and the Hospital Service*, English Universities Press: London

Macleod Clark, J. (1981) 'Communication in Nursing', *Nursing Times, 77*, 12-18

McFarlane, J. (1976) 'The Science and Art of Nursing', *Nursing Mirror*, 24 June, 64-6

Menzies, I. (1960) 'A Case Study of the Functioning of Social Systems as a Defence Against Anxiety', *Human Relations, 13*, 95-123

Rackham, N. and Morgan, T. (1971) *Behaviour Analysis in Training*, McGraw Hill: Maidenhead, Berks

Spence, S. and Shepherd, G. (1983) *Developments in Social Skills Training*, Academic Press: London

Stockwell, F. (1972) *The Unpopular Patient*, RCN: London

Sundeen, S.J., Stuart, G.W., Rankin, E. De S., and Cohen, S.A. (1981) *Nurse-Client Interaction*: Implementing the Nursing Process, Mosby: St Louis

Trower, P., Bryant, B. and Argyle, M. (1978) *Social Skills and Mental Health*, Methuen: London

Underwood, W.J. (1965) 'Evaluation of Laboratory Methods of Training', *Training Directors Journal, 19*, 24-40

van Ments, M. (1978) 'Role-Playing: Playing a Part or a Mirror to Meaning?' *Sagset Journal, 8*, 83-92

Williams, L.V. (1978) 'Patient Role-Play by Learners', *Nursing Times*, 4, 1402-6
Wilson-Barnett, J. (1978) 'Patients' Emotional Response to Barium X-Rays', *Journal of Advanced Nursing*, 3, 37-46

Useful Reading

Barker, D. (1980) *TA and Training*, Gower: Aldershot
Barker, L. (1971) *Listening Behavior*, Prentice Hall: Englewood Cliffs, New Jersey
Egan, G. (1975) *The Skilled Helper*, Brooks/Cole: California
Egan, G. (1976) *Interpersonal Living*, Brooks/Cole: California
Edwards, B.J. and Brilhart, J.K. (1981) *Communication in Nursing Practice*, C.V. Mosby: St. Louis
Garvin, C.D. (1981) *Contemporary Group Work*, Prentice Hall: Englewood Cliffs, New Jersey
Hays, J.S. and Larsen, K.H. (1963) *Interacting with Patients*, Macmillan: New York
Hein, E.C. (1980) *Communication in Nursing Practice*, Little, Brown and Company: Boston
Lange, S.P. (1978) 'Transactional Analysis and Nursing' in C.E. Carlson and B. Blackwell (eds) *Behavioral Concepts and Nursing Intervention*, J.B. Lippincott: Philadelphia
Miles, M.B. (1981) *Learning to Work in Groups*, Teachers College Press: New York
O'Brien, M.J. (1978) *Communications and Relationships in Nursing*, C.V. Mosby: St. Louis
Phillips, K. and Fraser, T. (1982) *The Management of Interpersonal Skills Training*, Gower: Aldershot
Rogers, C.R. (1961) *On Becoming a Person*, Houghton Mifflin: Boston
Satow, A. and Evans, M. (1983) *Working with Groups*, Tacade: Manchester
van Ments M. (1983) *The Effective use of Role-Play*, Kogan Page: London
Wiedenback, E. and Falls, C.E. (1978) *Communication: Key to Effective Nursing*, Tiresias Press: New York

13 ISSUES ARISING FROM TEACHING INTERPERSONAL SKILLS IN GENERAL NURSE TRAINING

Gary Marshfield

Introduction

The General Nursing Council syllabus for training (GNC, 1977) recommends that the 'nursing process' be adopted in the care of patients. Various models of the nursing process have been developed, ranging from those that incorporate biological, psychological and social aspects, to those that are based on the daily activities of living (Roper, 1980). Implicit in the recommendation to use the nursing process is that the nurse(s) should discover more information about the patient(s) in order to plan and execute their care. Whichever model of the nursing process is adopted, the assumption is that nurses will be competent in using communication or interpersonal skills. It is thus that a whole new area has been opened up for consideration by practitioners and educators of nursing alike. Recent research into the general field of communication in nursing (see, for example, reviews and projects presented by Faulkner, 1984) has identified several facets of interpersonal communication that may underlie patients' concern with the quality of the information and communication they receive in hospital (e.g. Ley, 1972; Reynolds, 1978; HMSO, 1979). The evidence that nurses relate superficially to patients, often using defensive or evasive verbal and non-verbal strategies, is incontrovertible (for example, Ashworth, 1980, 1984; Macleod Clark, 1981, 1984) but does not necessarily mean they *lack* interpersonal skills. Rather, it may well be that conversations with patients, their relatives and friends can elicit emotional reactions in the nurse(s) which inhibit their effective use of skill. Other chapters in this book consider this possibility further. (See, for example, those by Peter Banister and Carolyn Kagan (3), Ann Faulkner (4), Mark Burton (5), Desmond Cormack (7) and Carolyn Kagan (15).)

There is a growing interest in developing interpersonal skills aspects of general nurse training (see chapters by Jill Macleod Clark (1) and Ann Faulkner (16)). This chapter is concerned with the opportunities that can be made in general nurse training to explore specific interpersonal techniques, and to try to identify some of the problems that could occur for students, patients, teachers and colleagues as this element of nurse training develops. My comments are based on my experience of introducing and developing a 'communication' course into general nurse training at the Brighton School of Nursing over the last three years.

The Nature of Interpersonal Relationships

When *you* enter into an interpersonal relationship with someone else, have you ever considered just what is involved? It might be helpful for you to consider how relationships evolve, with reference to the following questions:

> How much did you, personally, select the person with whom you were to have the relationship?

> What kinds of biases and prejudices were operating during the inception of the relationship?

> Were there class, cultural or religious factors that influenced your decision to begin the relationship?

It must be obvious from reflecting on these questions that the initiation and establishment of most interpersonal relationships is a highly selective, time consuming and complex activity. However, when nurses encounter patients for the first time, the process is contracted, and they cannot choose whether or not to relate: they must embark upon their relationship immediately. From their own life experiences, nurses may well have the skills of initiating relationships, but may lack specific perceptual, observational and assessment skills that will enable them to establish therapeutic relationships with patients.

The Identification of Patient Needs

It is only through meaningful interaction between patients and nurses that patients' problems can be ascertained, and it is the nurses' responsibility to create the climate where these can be assessed. Interpersonal skill is necessary to identify three different dimensions of patients' needs that have implications for nursing care. These dimensions can be categorised into (1) *biological needs* — is the patient short of breath because of a disease process? (2) *psychological needs* — is the patient able to accept alteration of body image following stoma surgery? (3) *social needs* — is the single-parent patient concerned about who is to manage her/his children while s/he is in hospital?

If these needs are not met, anxiety may be aroused in the patient, which can have a detrimental effect on recovery. Indeed, Hayward's (1975) research indicates that if appropriate information is given to patients about their illness, then the amount of pain reported will decrease. It is this general *ability to meet patients' needs for information about their illness, nursing procedures and after-care* that I consider to be the purpose of interpersonal skills training and communication techniques teaching.

The Scope of Interpersonal Skill in Nursing

It is the professional responsibility of both qualified and student nurses to provide an environment in which therapeutic relationships with patients can be established and develop within a limited time scale. To enable this process to evolve, nurses require specific knowledge, skills and attitudes related to both sociological and psychological aspects of human interaction. This knowledge should include an understanding of the effects of illness on the psychological state of an individual, and of how this changed state may affect her/his ability (or inclination) to communicate with members of the health care team. In addition, knowledge regarding the significance of verbal and non-verbal behaviour and how this can influence patients' own behaviour is required. Specifically, the *skills* of (a) interpreting patients' verbal and non-verbal messages; (b) recognising signs of anxiety, distress, fear and misunderstanding; (c) helping patients overcome the difficulties presented by cultural or social class differences; and (d) developing awareness of how personal attitudes and prejudices influence others' behaviour, and of becoming aware of the extent that own needs, skills and attitudes can be used to block or encourage communication with others, are all prerequisites of effective, and therapeutic relationships.

The Interpersonal Nature of Nursing Care

However nursing care is organised, nurses will always be able to offer a special relationship to individual patients that will bring their interpersonal skills into operation, and it is this special quality that I believe to be the essence of interpersonal skill that benefits patients and influences their prognoses. Because it is difficult to define or pin down the properties of individual nurses' relationships with individual patients, it is also difficult to measure the quality or effectiveness of such relationships. However, the initial identification of patients' care needs, and the evaluation of the extent to which these needs may be met, goes some way to making such an assessment. In addition, tutors can help students evaluate their own interpersonal relationships through shared observation of the interactive elements in the procedure, with some analysis of the situation from the students, their supervisors or the patients themselves. (See chapters by Peter Banister and Carolyn Kagan (3), Ann Faulkner (16), and Bill Reynolds, (14) for further discussion of the issues involved in the measurement of the quality of interpersonal relationships.)

Taking all these considerations into account, it should be clear that some time devoted to interpersonal skills in basic nurse training would be time well spent. Indeed the importance of teaching interpersonal skills to student nurses is now being recognised for two reasons. Firstly, researchers such as Hayward (1975), Boore (1978), Wilson-Barnett (1978) and Macleod Clark (1981) have clearly demonstrated specific and general deficits in the interpersonal skills of nurses. Secondly, recent syllabi of training imply a care delivery format that will demand greater emphasis on nurse-patient interaction. This has obvious implications for nurse educators who will have to consider changes to their (traditional) teaching sessions and methods.

Interpersonal Skills in the Context of General Nurse Training

If I am going to teach student nurses interpersonal skills while they are undergoing a three year general nurse training programme, I am faced with the mutually dependent questions illustrated in Figure 13.1. Ideally, the whole teaching team should review the entire three year curriculum, in order to assess where interpersonal skill input could be usefully added to theoretical input. I have found, for instance, that the basic psychology component taught previously has overlapped with communication skills: teaching time can thus be saved by restructuring sessions. The incorporation of interpersonal skills does not necessarily mean *additional* teaching, but rather implies re-evaluation of other teaching sessions. After all, interpersonal skill is integral to nursing care and not a separate 'subject' or focus area.

Figure 13.1: Issues to Consider on Introducing
Interpersonal Skills to Basic Nurse Training

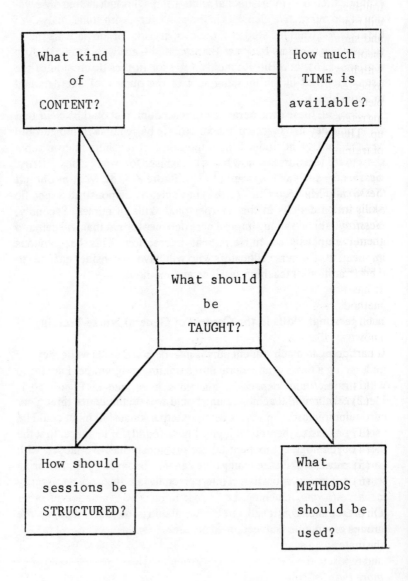

Content of Interpersonal Skills Training

A summary of the type of content I use during the first 18 months of training is given below. (See Table 13.1.) I anticipate that each session will require at least two hours, and that experiential exercises, role-play and simulations will be included in each session. There will also be theoretical background to the sessions, and students will be provided with handouts summarising the session content. Students will also be expected to undertake some reading and produce some work, completed during their own time, in relation to some of the sessions. Reading references will be provided, and students encouraged to follow them up. Thus, there are a total of 15 sessions during the first 18 months of training:

Sessions 1 and 2 are an introduction to communication;
Sessions 3-8 are elements of communication and include micro-skills training;
Sessions 9-15 involve putting together the micro-skills and applying them to nursing practice.

Teaching/Learning Methods

It has proved most useful to use experiential teaching and learning methods (see chapter 12, by Anne Tomlinson, for full discussion of such techniques). I favour a method that liberally employs what are known as 'trigger materials' — anything that 'triggers' the discussion of a particular aspect or topic. Examples of such triggers might be:

(1) role play situations;
(2) captured video material of an individual or nurse patient interaction;
(3) professional articles;
(4) patients' own perceptions of the hospitalisation experience;
(5) pictures of either patients or nurses;
(6) audio or written transcripts of patients' interactions.

On presenting 'trigger' material, either to the class as a whole, to small groups of students or to each individually, students will either discuss the material in a large group or work on selected aspects of the situation and report to the large group. I have found the large group should be *no more than 14* students. The method of choice for an individual group really needs to rest with the particular tutor who is running that session; if a student member is running the session then s/he should be guided by the tutor as to what sort of session content to include.

Table 13.1: The Content of Interpersonal Skills Training Sessions

---

SESSION 1: The Place, Importance and Relevance of Communication in Nursing
An introduction to communication, human needs, health education and the skills required for effective communication. Understanding self and others. Attitudes, culture and class variables.

SESSION 2: Elements of Communication
Verbal and non-verbal components of communication. Micro-skills defined. Explanation of ways to improve them.

SESSION 3: Listening and Attending Behaviours
Listening habits, hearing, recognising cues. Improved skill in listening, iden-tifying cues, practising skills.

SESSION 4: Questioning
Obtaining information. Assessing patients. Types of questions and informa-tion likely to be gained from each type. Exploring feelings.

SESSION 5: Reinforcing and Encouraging
Verbal and non-verbal encouragement. Praise, valuing, repeating and reflecting.

SESSION 6: Information Giving
The purpose of giving information. Facilitating and inhibiting the passage of information. Principles of effective information transmission.

SESSION 7: Openings, Control of Interaction, Closings
Effective openings. Time and environmental restrictions. Successful and appropriate control of conversations. Effective closings. Feelings and behaviour.

SESSION 8: Comfort and Reassurance
Patient centred behaviour. Nurse centred behaviour. Relationship formation, purpose and benefit. Constructing barriers. Research. Health Education.

SESSION 9: Combining Micro-skills and Applying them to Patient Care
Assessing a patient, and relatives' needs for communication. Relationship to the nursing process. Appropriate nursing behaviour. Admission of a patient. Problem-solving, goals.

SESSION 10: Communicating with Other Members of the Health Care Team
Authority, power and control, roles. Attitudes. Organisations. Accountability assertion and patient advocacy.

SESSION 11: Nursing a Dying Patient
Diagnosis. Defence. Denial. Detachment. Death and the dying process. Trust. Empathy. Sharing. Identification and self-awareness.

SESSION 12: Preparing a Patient for Discharge
Health promotion. The nurse as a teacher. Patients' rights. Education aims.
Alcoholism. Heart disease. Stoma care. Smoking.

SESSION 13: Nursing and Communicating with Geriatric and Stroke Patients
Defining inhibiting factors. Physiological failure of sight, hearing, smell, taste,
touch, movement. Frustration, anger, rejection.

SESSION 14: Communicating with Patients before and after Surgery
Pre and post-operative care. Research findings. Identifying fear. Anxiety and
recovery. Reducing anxiety.

SESSION 15: Investigations on Surgical and Medical Patients
Verbal and non-verbal skills and strategies providing a framework for
effective communication with patients and colleagues. How to encourage
effective communication with 'difficult ', confused', 'anxious', and 'depressed'
patients.

Videotapes are particularly valuable 'triggers', and there are several commercially available tapes showing nurses in a wide variety of care settings, interacting with patients. The tapes can be purchased or hired by the education division. The scenarios can be viewed without sound to enable students to focus on non-verbal behaviour and its implications, or with sound, in order to compare verbal and non-verbal effects. Discussion of the situation provides students with an opportunity to explore options available in a variety of situations and perhaps recognise that some strategies are more appropriate than others.

As an adjunct to the 'triggers', the tutor needs adequate library resources to be available so that students can take tapes to review them there. Thus cassette machines should be available. Students also need access to quite a wide variety of nursing, sociology and psychology books, and again it is quite helpful, at the end of each session to summarise the main learning objectives of the session together with additional reading that the students may or may not wish to undertake. There is no point in recommending that students follow up references that are not available in the library.

I have found that it is very important to have access to a wide variety of teaching aids including video-tape material, video monitoring facilities, slides, photocopying and stencilling facilities, as I need a multi-faceted approach to demonstrate interpersonal skills. de Tournyay (1971) supports the notion that if the teacher is trying to stimulate the students' emotional and cognitive development then a non-didactic method of teaching is appropriate; so, using a wide variety of teaching aids will be advantageous.

If the school itself has its own video recorder and is fortunate enough to have a camera, it is possible to go into the ward and make your own video tapes of clinical situations, etc. The great problem with this is that you probably don't have film making skills! I have also found it useful just to go into a ward area and take photographs of nurses in nursing situations and show the pictures to the students and ask them what they think is happening here, what might the nurse be saying etc. In this way students can actually look at the non-verbal behaviour of the individuals, albeit in static form. This raises ethical issues, however. The film makers need to be aware of the difficulties of gaining permission from patients and nurses involved. The participants need to be sure that the material will be used for educational purposes, and who the audience will be. They must have the right to withdraw permission if they so wish. I like to show the material that I have filmed to the staff, together with the patient, in order to identify potential problems in using the material. This is difficult if either party has left the hospital! Most patients do, however, wish to help students learn, and are often pleased to be introduced on film.

The Learning Context

The environment for teaching interpersonal skills needs to be warm, spacious, and to be a comfortable setting in an area where emotions and feelings can be expressed. Nursing students may wish to talk loudly, shout, argue, dispute or feel sad. The noise that may be created could interrupt formalised teaching sessions, and if the participants are aware of the effects of the sound effects of their session on other classes it could have an inhibiting effect. Adler, Rosenfeld and Towne (1980) state that the 'climate' i.e. physical location of rooms where interpersonal work is occurring is important as it can influence the performance of the group. Think of how variations in weather can influence how you feel and act; in a similar vein, the environment for teaching must be considered by the teachers. Colleagues may object to noise/disruption caused to their teaching by those engaging in interpersonal skills work. If the whole teaching team is involved in re-vamping the curriculum, this reaction will be minimised.

Students' Experiences of Interpersonal Skills Learning

Students often say that they are not sure what they have learnt during interpersonal skills sessions. In general, they perceive their learning to be directly related to having a 'wodge of notes'. Abercrombie (1974) however, shows clearly that interpersonal skills learning may not occur immediately; indeed, it may take upwards of two years, in so far as it may be an evolving and developing thing for the learner. Giving the students a handout perhaps minimises their anxiety that they may not have any *information* content about the session.

The students' personal evaluation of the sessions provides the teacher with feedback, and examples of their comments may assist future planning of content of sessions.

I have received evaluations of sessions which clearly demonstrate that learners' sensitivity, insight and perceptions are developing. Examples come in the form of written evaluations, poems or verbal feedback:

> I particularly enjoyed communication although it is difficult to define how valuable it has been. However it has made me aware of things.

> Communication discussions valuable.

> The videos in communications make the nurse more observant.

> Discussions in communications were often interesting — helpful as the group got to know each other.

WHOSE TIME

A row of silent, staring faces,
Greet my eyes,
Their time simply their own
Not mine; on this day
For them the minds of timelessness
Slip into a fathomless jigsaw dream
Of lifelong memories, experiences all untold —
Through mirrored visions of hazy past,
And laced with glimpses not long, to last
This moment now, this reality?
It brings to my mind this movement of time

Which comes and goes and never stays
So who's to say
Where is the reality?

This poem was submitted by a learner in response to the question 'How did communication skills teaching help you to understand elderly patients?'

For educational purposes, however, there may be a need to attempt more formal assessment of student learning. I have found that, following interpersonal skills sessions, students answering nursing care questions demonstrate a wider range of perceptiveness and sensitivity. After participating in interpersonal skills sessions students included the following recommendations (in order of importance) in answer to the question *'How would a nurse deal with a situation where a patient is withdrawn?'*

Communicate with patient
Provide diversion, books etc.

Nurse should be non-threatening
Nurse should be calm and soothing

Nurse should provide security
Nurse should show kindness

Give patients time, sit with them, stay close, touch, hold, show friendliness

Provide constant supervision

Encourage patient to take interest in the environment

Be prepared to remove patient from surroundings

Be a guide to relatives

Make sure patient is comfortable (physically)

Go to patient frequently

These answers demonstrate a wide range of alternatives, based broadly on interpersonal considerations. Students who had not undergone interpersonal skills sessions were not able to generate such a wide range of options. Of course, *knowing* of alternatives is no guarantee that the students would be able to put them into effective practice. However, as Carolyn Kagan (Chapter 15) points out, interpersonal *knowledge* is a necessary component of interpersonal *skill*.

It is also important to point out that students frequently comment on the fact that some sessions are tiring, and that they experience feelings of self-consciousness. Some sessions make them relive and feel experiences, and sometimes this causes them pain. However, they do say that if they are able to talk out their feelings with a member of the group privately, or individually with the tutor running the sessions, the seemingly negative effects often have positive outcomes. It is essential that the opportunities for personal support are available, and this has implications for the skills required by interpersonal skills teachers.

Implications for Nurse Tutors

The training for interpersonal skills and communication techniques is beginning to be included as part of Teachers of Nursing courses. This is a recent innovation, and there will be teachers who would wish to acquire training and experience in these methods because they had not been part of their own teachers' course. Hopefully, the statutory 're-fresher' week that all nurse teachers are obligated to attend after five years' teaching experience could have interpersonal skills techniques included in the content. This would give some respectability to interpersonal skill as an integral part of nurse education.

If tutors are committed to interactive, experiential and experimental learning methods, they may in fact have a major attitudinal problem with their colleagues, who may challenge the value and the purpose of this teaching. Such interpersonal 'conflict' created amongst the tutors may be detrimental to a particular tutor who is trying to develop innovative and creative methods of interpersonal skills teaching.

Interpersonal skill issues are accorded little professional credibility, as they are rarely acknowledged by nurse tutors when they appear in answers to formal examinations or in the assessment of nursing skill. Furthermore, the examining bodies place greater emphasis on other areas of knowledge such as, say, disordered physiology. I suppose that it is the old argument that if nurses do not understand the normal cardiac physiology, they will not understand heart disease and this can be catastrophic for the patients' nursing care. However, if the patients feel the attitudes of the nurses are 'off-putting', or judgemental, and that they do not demonstrate empathy and rapport with them, they may choose not to disclose information to the nurses that could have equally catastrophic results.

A good example of this occurred recently. A patient informed me he was on a particular drug for depressive illness that would seriously have interacted with the medication he was receiving for pain in his back. When asked why he had not told the doctor and nurses about this he replied, 'I did not want them to think that I was neurotic. They do when people have pains in the back'! Emotionally, this patient had a vast amount of personal information to give, some relevant and some irrelevant to his current admission. He thought we might judge him by what he had disclosed. If this patient's experience is to have any meaning for nurses, then training needs to encourage the development of self-awareness and sensitivity to the *whole* communication process. It is only with training that student and qualified nurses will learn to elicit and use personal information therapeutically.

All general nurses have a responsibility to develop their interpersonal skills, and the Schools of Nursing have a responsibility to provide the opportunities for them to do so.

Summary and Conclusions

On considering the introduction of interpersonal skills to general nurse training courses, several issues are inevitably raised (see Table 13.2).

Table 13.2: Summary of Issues Pertaining to the Introduction of Interpersonal Skills to General Nurse Training

ETHICAL ISSUES
    Patients' rights and privacy
    Students' rights and privacy

VALIDITY ISSUES
    Personal growth for learners
    Attitudinal assessment (including ward reports)
    Perceptiveness and sensitivity to patient needs
    Improvement in patient care

TEACHING
    Content
    Methods
    Resources
    Facilities

TUTORS
    Training
    Acceptance
    Resources

SUPPORT SYSTEMS
    Students
    Tutors
    Colleagues

Furthermore, there will be inherent problems in any attempt to change the process of nursing, whether it be of practice or training. Open and honest discussion between members of the health care team, between health professionals and patients and between students and tutors and ward staff will be required. Only then will problems be aired and workable solutions be effected.

From my experience of introducing interpersonal skills to general nurse training, several themes need emphasising.

(1) Exploration of the ethical issues in tutorial meetings means that participants are aware of some of the pitfalls likely to occur, and to find suitable options to prevent their occurrence.

(2) The personal growth and motivation of the students is a naturally evolving process. I have found that the responsibility of a greater involvement with patients means students have to have thought about the responsibility of creating therapeutic relationships with patients. I consider that the illness process, with its biological, psychological, sociological and cultural impact, requires nurses to reflect upon their own values.

(3) The required attitudinal changes in nursing students need to be monitored at the end of each period of clinical practice (possibly in the form of the ward report). This should indicate how the nurses are developing their sensitivity and perceptiveness to meet the emotional, psychological and practical care needs of the patients.

(4) The heads of training schools, who control the budgets, will have to be committed to expenditure on a wider range of learning resource material than previously to allow the tutors to operate effectively, and meet the learners' needs of handouts, text books, films and video cassettes.

(5) The nurse teaching profession will need to ask for courses and training schemes in order that tutors without interpersonal/communication skills training can acquire these skills before commencing modules within the three-year training programme.

(6) The provision of either a formal or informal support system for both the students and their teachers is desirable. To date, this has appeared for the teachers in the form of an Interpersonal Skills group that initially met nationally, and currently meets locally. At these meetings we exchange ideas, give support for peers who develop new packages, and meet like-minded people; it has certainly proved invaluable to members. Similar schemes could be offered to students.

Despite all the difficulties, the profession must have a commitment to interpersonal/communication skills teaching in nurse education and practice. We must enable both ourselves and patients to feel comfortable in the nurse-patient relationship. Only then will patients receive the benefits of modern technology, *and* of the psychosocial support necessary to effect recovery, palliation of illness or a peaceful death. This is the essence of good nursing care.

References

Abercrombie M.L.J. (1974) *The Anatomy of Judgement*, Penguin: Harmondsworth

Adler, R.B. Rosenfeld, L.B., and Towne, N. (1980) *Interplay*, Holt, Rinehart and Winston : London

Ashworth, P. (1980) *Care to Communicate*, Royal College of Nursing : London

Ashworth, P. (1984) 'Communicating in an Intensive Care Unit' in A. Faulkner (ed.), *Recent Advances in Nursing* : 7, *Communication*, Churchill Livingstone : Edinburgh

Boore, J. (1978) *A Prescription for Recovery*, Royal College of Nursing : London

Faulkner, A. (ed.) (1984) *Recent Advances in Nursing* : 7, *Communication*, Churchill Livingstone : Edinburgh

GNC (1977) *General Nursing Syllabus for Training*, General Nursing Council : London

Hayward, J. (1975) *Information — A Prescription Against Pain*, Royal College of Nursing : London

HMSO (1979) Health Services Commissioner — *Annual Report of Session 1978-79*, HMSO : London

Ley, P. (1972) 'Complaints Made by Hospital Staff and Patients : A review of the literature', *Bulletin of British Psychological Society*, 25, 115-20

Macleod Clark, J. (1981) 'Nurse-Patient Communication', *Nursing Times*, 77, 12-18

Macleod Clark, J. (1984) 'Verbal Communication in Nursing' in A. Faulkner (ed.), *Recent Advances in Nursing* : 7, *Communication*, Churchill Livingstone : Edinburgh

Reynolds, M. (1978) 'No News is Bad News : Patients' views about communication in hospital', *British Medical Journal*, 1, 1673-6

Roper, N. (1980) *The Elements of Nursing*, Churchill Livingstone : Edinburgh

de Tournyay, R. (1971) *Strategies in Teaching Nursing*, Wiley : London

Wilson-Barnett, J. (1978) 'Patients' Emotional Responses to Barium X-rays', *Journal of Advanced Nursing*, 3, 37-46

Further Reading

Argyle, M. (1975) *Bodily Communication*, Methuen : London

Argyle, M. (1982) *The Psychology of Interpersonal Behaviour* (4th edn) Penguin : London

Berne, E. (1976) *Games People Play*, Penguin : London

Edwards, B.J. and Brilhart, J.K. (1981) *Communication in Nursing Practice*, Mosby : St. Louis

Hein, E.C. (1980) *Communication in Nursing Practice*, Little, Brown and Company : Boston

Knapp, M.L. (1972) *Non-Verbal Communication in Human Interaction*, Holt, Rinehart and Winston : New York

O'Brien J. (1978) *Communications and Relationships in Nursing*, Mosby : St. Louis

Rogers, C. (1961) *On Becoming a Person*, Houghton Mifflin : Boston

Satir, V. (1972) *Peoplemaking*, Science and Behaviour Books, Inc. : California

Smith, V.M. and Bass, T.A. (1982) *Communication for the Health Care Team* (UK adaptation by A. Faulkner) Harper and Row : London

Sundeen, S.J., Stuart, G.W., Rankin, E. de S. and Cohen, S.A. (1981) *Nurse-Client Interaction : Implementing the Nursing Process*, Mosby : St. Louis

Tschudin, V. (1982) *Counselling Skills for Nurses*, Balliere Tindall : London

14 ISSUES ARISING FROM TEACHING INTERPERSONAL SKILLS IN PSYCHIATRIC NURSE TRAINING

Bill Reynolds

Introduction

One of the major therapeutic tools available to psychiatric nurses is the constructive use of interpersonal skills (IPS) (Altschul, 1972; Cormack, 1976). Thus the teaching of IPS forms the basis, in one form or another, for much of psychiatric nurse training. In this chapter I will be concerned with some of the issues that make this task particularly daunting, but at the same time challenging and exciting. Many of these issues are common to all fields of nursing, but some are particular because of the special nature of psychiatric nursing. I shall base my discussion on my experience over the years of teaching psychiatric nurse students at the Highland College of Nursing at Inverness, and will give examples throughout of how we have attempted to confront some of the blocks to effective teaching/learning. I must say, though, that what follows reflects the stage we have reached to date: we ourselves are continually learning, as teachers, and adapting our techniques and methods in the light of our (and our students') experiences.

In the course of the chapter, I will discuss some of the barriers to teaching IPS to psychiatric nurse students, and some techniques we have introduced to try to overcome them. I shall go on to use the teaching/learning of counselling skills as an example of how we incorporate the need to develop self-awareness and empathic abilities in students, if they are to make constructive, therapeutic use of IPS. Finally, I shall consider the nature of the student-teacher relationship that must be created if self-awareness and interpersonal skills are to be confronted openly and non-defensively by students and teachers alike.

Barriers to Teaching

Psychiatric nursing has for a long time been an extremely difficult subject to teach. Part of the explanation for this difficulty lies in the fact

228

that diverse opinions exist, at least in the United Kingdom, about what psychiatric nurses do, or should do. Some of this role confusion may be related to the different approaches towards the treatment of mental illness. For example, the medical model of care views the client as a passive host of disease, and a non-participating recipient of treatment, while the social model of care views the client as an individual who is responsible to varying degrees for his/her own actions, and emphasises the therapeutic value of the daily interpersonal experiences occurring between staff and clients, within a therapeutic milieu. The medical model tends to prescribe a protective role for the nurse, while both humanistic and social models prescribe a counselling or psychotherapeutic role for the nurse. Whatever the model, it is assumed that constructive use of interpersonal skills will be therapeutic.

In spite of the fact that both the United States and United Kingdom nursing literature has prescribed a counselling role for the psychiatric nurse, several writers have suggested that United Kingdom nurses have poor role clarity. Research based studies have also demonstrated that there is a considerable difference between the role prescribed for the psychiatric nurse in the literature, and the observed role. Cormack (1976) demonstrated that while many clients did value conversations with a nurse, observations of nurses at work suggested that their main purpose in interacting with clients was to gather clinical data relating to the clients' symptoms, not to influence these symptoms. Ferguson (1978) suggested that there was serious confusion about the role and function of the psychiatric nurse, not least perhaps, because psychiatric nurses have often claimed that psychiatric nursing was 'common sense', and that nurses frequently did not have an easily identifiable perspective to guide them in their dealings with problematic situations (Altschul 1972). Caine and Smail (1968) appear to support Altschul's observations, when they claim that the psychiatric nurse's attitude to his/her work must be determined by a complex interaction between his/her own personality and beliefs, the biases of those responsible for his/her training, and the general atmosphere and ideology of the hospital in which he/she works. Consequently it is argued that in order to teach psychiatric nursing effectively, the teacher must know how nurses can contribute to the overall care of patients, what skills and knowledge are essential and how to help the student to apply theoretical principles to practice.

A second major difficulty faced by teachers in this field lies in the fact that they are rarely practising nurses, and may have limited contact with the clinical areas. This fact may be of greater significance in psychiatric nursing than in other fields due to the interpersonal nature of the nurses' work. Interpersonal behaviours which involve the use of verbal communication and body language are often referred to as *low visibility* skills because they are more difficult to teach, observe and assess than technical skills, such as administering oral medication, or physical care, such as bathing a client. It is possible that the ability of the student to recognise interpersonal behaviour and its effect is dependent upon the development of a non-threatening working relationship between the teacher and student, which cannot be developed or fully utilised in the classroom alone.

It can be argued that low visibility skills such as psychotherapeutic communication take longer to establish than physical or technical skills. Davis (personal communication, 1981) and Melia (1981) indicated that learners often find it difficult to talk to clients about their illness, treatment or personal problems. Reynolds, too (1982) has noted that learners found it difficult to respond to clients' direct questions with needed facts, to discuss feelings with the client, or to help the clients to focus on areas of concern, during the progress of a psychiatric nursing module. It is suggested that the intensive presence of the teacher on the wards is required to provide students with role modelling, direction, and interpretation during clinical experience. It may well be that it is the practice of nursing followed by analyses of its effect, that influences the students' behaviour and role clarity.

It is for these reasons that I suggest that it is unfortunate that nurse teachers in the United Kingdom have become predominantly classroom based, have ceased to practise nursing, and have largely delegated responsibility for the supervision of students in the clinical areas to practising nurses. Practising nurses may not have teaching skills, or the time or motivation to teach; they may not share the teachers' perception of the nurse's role: for example if they do not see counselling as being a primary function, it is unlikely that the students will observe or practise counselling, unless their teacher is actually present. I would suggest therefore, that it is essential for all teachers to be engaged in practical psychiatric nursing with their students in order to demonstrate skills, and to provide the prolonged direction, support and analysis that helps students to develop interpersonal skills and to understand their clinical experiences more fully. (Of course, this assumes that the teachers will present 'good' role models!)

A further problem faced by United Kingdom teachers is that the number of research based studies relevant to psychiatric nursing is still very limited. Even so, Boore (1984) notes that nurse educators are rarely 'research minded' and seem reluctant to base their teaching on research findings. It is my view that unless the emphasis on nursing research is increased, we will remain a discipline that relies on other professionals to suggest to us what we ought to be doing for our clients. We will continue to work by intuition and to be influenced by our favourite textbook or anecdotes from the past. Research will enable us to develop nursing theory and to identify nursing interventions which are the most effective in helping clients to regain the optimum level of health. In other words, research will tell us what psychiatric nursing is.

The Problem Oriented, Behavioural Approach

It is suggested that the most effective way of teaching psychiatric nursing is to use an approach which enables students to focus attention on specific nursing problems that the clients present, to prescribe and implement nursing interventions, and to measure the effectiveness of these. Notice that I have emphasised nursing diagnosis and nursing care prescriptions. Medical diagnosis and medical care prescriptions are relevant to the nature of the nurses' role, but they do not necessarily focus on the phenomena which nurses treat. Reynolds and Cormack (1982, p.233) have stated that the medical model does not always provide nurses with a clear idea of their reasons for providing nursing care. They demonstrated the problem in the following manner:

> One patient with a diagnosis of 'chronic schizophrenia, undifferentiated type' may present problems relating to dependence and low self esteem, or to psychomotor skills and anxiety, or to reality (perception) and trust.

Clearly there is a wide range of variation in the nursing needs of individuals who share the same medical diagnosis. It can be argued that if nurses were not aware of specific nursing needs, they would not know if their responses towards their clients were appropriate or not, and would not be aware of the existence of problems which were within the scope of nurses to treat. The potential problems identified in the example given, such as trust or low self esteem, and their consequences for the client, for example, a tendency to isolate him/herself, or to be hostile towards others, require nursing diagnosis and intervention. It is suggested that a problem orientated enquiry into the needs of our clients will

Figure 14.1: The Learner's Daily Activity Guide: Side 1

STUDENT'S NAME: _____

DATE: _____

INITIALS OF CLIENT WHOM YOU INTEND TO INTERACT WITH TODAY: _____

CLIENT'S NURSING NEEDS

PSYCHOLOGICAL PROBLEMS	YES	NO
Reality Problems		
Affect Problems		
Trust Problems		
Hostility Problems		
Social Skills		
Self Esteem Problems		
Dependency Problems		

PHYSICAL PROBLEMS	YES	NO

SOCIAL PROBLEMS	YES	NO

DESCRIPTION OF CLIENT'S PROBLEMS

DESCRIPTION OF GOALS FOR TODAY'S
INTERACTION

SELF GOALS (Nursing Approaches)	CLIENT GOALS (What the client does)

Figure 14.2: The Learner's Daily Activity Guide: Side 2

DESCRIPTION OF STUDENT'S BEHAVIOUR DURING INTERACTION

		YES	NO
1	Purposeful activity		
2	Uses +ve/-ve reinforcement		
3	" eye contact		
4	" physical contact		
5	" postural echo		
6	" displays genuineness		
7	" tolerates frustration		
8	" therapeutic counselling techniques		

EVALUATION OF INTERACTION

		YES	NO
1	Facilitated assessment of client's mental state		
2	Client's situation or environment altered		
3	Client's behaviour altered		
4	Useful in initiating a relationship		

help to answer the question, 'What do nurses treat?' The focus will then be on the caring functions of the nurse, which are distinct from, but complementary to, the caring functions of the physician.

The Learner's Daily Activity Guide

In response to the question, 'What do nurses treat?' and to help learners to plan and evaluate nursing care, teachers at the Highland College of Nursing, Inverness, have introduced this teaching tool (see Figure 14.1 and Figure 14.2). The tool is used by students and teachers, at a daily pre-clinical and post-clinical conference, held during the clinical component of a psychiatric nursing module. The same teachers provide students with their classroom teaching and with supervision during a significant period of their clinical experience (10 days). The first page (Figure 14.1) is completed by the student and forms the basis of the pre-clinical conference between student and teacher. Discussion focuses on the student's ability/inability to identify and to describe clients' needs in measurable behavioural terms, and to describe both self goals (what the nurse does), and client goals (what the client will achieve), in measurable behavioural terms. Sometimes the student's observations and goals can also be discussed with the client, and they form the basis and focus for some of the nursing care which the student will deliver that day. Examples of nursing care include initiating informal discussion groups, or sharing activities with the client such as baking, playing Scrabble or shopping. During these student-initiated activities teachers fully participate and act as role models. The second page of this tool (Figure 14.2) is completed by the teacher during a post-clinical conference with the student. During this conference the student and teacher focus on the content of the interaction being discussed. In particular, an attempt is made to describe interpersonal behaviours such as the use of body language. Finally, an evaluation is made of the effects of the interaction on the client's needs, and an assessment is made of the appropriateness of the student's goals.

The daily activity guide provides focus and structure to an intensive client-centred clinical teaching programme, and provides valuable clues about students' ability to identify nursing needs, to evaluate the effect of care and to identify the interpersonal behaviours of both student and teacher. In addition it emphasises that psychiatric nursing is a specific and therapeutic activity built on behavioural concepts and delivered within a holistic framework.

Teaching and Learning Interpersonal Skills

The Counselling Role of the Nurse

It has long been argued that the emphasis in psychiatric nursing should be on the counselling role. Peplau (1960) stressed the importance of verbal interactions in the formation of therapeutic relationships. Peplau (1962) also defined the specialist psychiatric nurse as a clinical specialist in interpersonal techniques. This view is subscribed to by many others, such as Ministry of Health Report (1968) and Nicol and Withington (1981). Whether psychiatric nursing should adopt a counselling framework, or whether counselling skills should be viewed as part of the psychiatric nurse's repertoire of therapeutic skills, the learning of counselling skills will be a legitimate part of basic psychiatric nurse training. I will use the teaching/learning of counselling skills as a 'case study' to illustrate many of the issues that arise with regard to the teaching/learning of any interpersonal skill(s) in psychiatric settings.

Recorded Nurse-Client Interactions

In an attempt to help students to develop an awareness of basic counselling skills and to integrate college theory with practice, teachers at the Highland College have included recorded clinical interviews as a component of the students' clinical teaching programme. This strategy was described by Reynolds (1982), and has now been extended to include all students during their first psychiatric nursing module.

The recorded interaction consists of six private interviews between the student and client, lasting for thirty minutes. A contract is formed between the student and client which involves an agreement about confidentiality, content, time and individual responsibility. The client is invited to talk about her/himself as a person, and both participants agree to attend, or to inform the other if they are unable to attend the interview for any reason. During the scheduled thirty minutes verbatim notes are recorded by the student of all verbal interaction occurring between the nurse and the client, and a record is made of the client's non-verbal communication. These notes include the student's personal feelings relating to the situation. The notes are made available for later discussion, during a student-teacher meeting, but are otherwise regarded as completely confidential. During the interviews students attempt to practise psychotherapeutic techniques practised in college, such as responding to direct questions with needed facts, asking open questions and conveying empathy towards the client. The student also experiences, and learns how to respond to, many problems presented by the client and resulting from the milieu which hinder the development of the helping relationship. Examples of problems include non-attendance at interview, coping with silence, or to delusional ideation.

The following evaluation tool is used by Inverness teachers at the post-clinical conference which follows the student's interview, (see Figures 14.3 and 14.4).

The Rationale for Recording Clinical Interviews. If communication strategies which are an integral part of the counselling role are to be learned, both the student and teacher need clinical data that tell us whether the language of the nurse is constructive or destructive. Physicians are guided by clinical data in the form of laboratory reports and other measurements such as electronic blood pressure recordings. The problem in nurse-client verbal interactions is the ambiguity of the data. You have to make it more concrete, in the sense that you hold it still while you look at it.

Most students in my experience have claimed that they can accurately remember the content of nurse-client verbal interactions, but studies conducted with crime victims, and tape recorded checks, conducted with students in the United States, have demonstrated that the recall is not accurate. Peplau (personal communication, 1983) noted that students nearly always change the data to make themselves look better. I have observed that, when there is no record of the verbal interaction, my own students have tended to describe what the client has said, but rarely described their own language. In a further communication Peplau (personal communication, 1983), stated that most psychiatric illness is reflected in the language of the client; if it is a thought disorder, the only way that this can be corrected or helped is by the language of the nurse interacting with the language of the client. Something the nurse says to the client and repeats regularly, can reinforce a thought disorder. This can only be detected and learned by recording the interaction and collecting raw data.

In my view raw data enable us to make inferences or judgements about the content of verbal interactions. The teacher is less concerned with whether particular students have done well or badly, but looks at the data objectively so that the students can begin to reshape what they are saying to the client. For example, students can learn if they are listening, being non-directive, neutral or genuine. If students are able to do this sufficiently often with their clients, the clients will experience a supportive and non-threatening relationship with their nurses. It is often claimed that nurses help their clients within the framework of a

Figure 14.3: Analysis of Recorded One-to-One Nurse Patient
Interaction : Side 1

LEARNERS NAME:

WARD:

DATE:

TIME:

INTERACTION NO:

		YES	NO	COMMENTS
1	Satisfactory Environment			
2	Avoided Frequent Direct Questions			
3	Avoided Value Judgements			
4	Listens carefully to the Patient			
5	Tolerates Silences			
6	Sought clarification on points not understood			
7	Helped the patient to focus on areas of concern			
8	Responded to direct questions with needed facts			
9	Attempted to develop an empathic understanding of the patient			
10	Conveyed empathy towards the patient when opportunity arose			
11	Terminated the interaction smoothly eg with an evaluation or future plan			
12	Responded well to specific problems presented by the patient during interaction eg Patient arrives late, remains silent, wants to extend time limits etc			

Figure 14.4: Analysis of Recorded One-to-One Nurse Patient
Interaction : Side 2

NURSING NEEDS REVEALED BY THE INTERACTION

EFFECTS OF THE INTERACTION ON THE PATIENT

therapeutic relationship. Kalkman (1967, p.226), when referring to the therapeutic relationship, described it in the following manner:

> ... a prolonged relationship between a nurse therapist and a client, during which the client can feel accepted by the nurse as a person of worth, feels free to express himself without fear of rejection or censure, and enables him to learn more satisfactory and productive patterns of behaviour.

Examples of behaviours which teachers should help students to practise include:

(a) asking open ended questions;

(b) resisting the temptation to lead when silence occurs;

(c) helping the client to focus on areas of concern;

(d) seeking clarification when the communicated message is unclear;

(e) responding to direct questions;

(f) reflecting the language of the client;

(g) conveying empathy in a manner which allows the client to refute the observation if it is inaccurate.

If the students are able to establish these behaviours on a regular basis, they will not only provide a counselling service to the clients, but will increase the potential for therapeutic relationships to develop.

Methods of Recording Clinical Interviews

There are different ways of collecting 'objective' data on the content of interviews, and methods of recording may include:

(a) verbatim notes during the interview;

(b) process recording immediately following the interview;

(c) audiotape and videotape recordings.

All of these methods have advantages and disadvantages, and range from the less objective to the more objective methods. Whichever method is used, students need to acquire accurate perceptual and observational skills. This is, in itself, no mean feat.

Verbatim Notes. The criticism levelled at verbatim notes is that they are unnatural and distracting, and may detract from the therapeutic process. It is difficult, even impossible, under certain circumstances to record the interaction in its entirety. I have observed, however, that with experience, most students become very adept at recording most of the content, and develop a competence which allows them to record only what is important or very significant. However, it is the very nuances that are missed that are often critical for the learning and development of skill. It has to be admitted that a minority of students do find this process very difficult, and it is often the students who are the most resistant who find it most difficult to record.

In spite of these difficulties I prefer to use verbatim notes with basic and inexperienced students. I believe that it is potentially useful for the students to have some raw data in front of them during practice. This provides them with some clues about how to respond; it allows them to slow down the interaction and to consider what the client has communicated to them. It also provides them with an opportunity to evaluate their own communication as it is occurring. Students often claim that when they read their own communication they become aware of inappropriate verbal responses or missed opportunities. For example they may have failed to listen or make an empathic statement at an appropriate moment.

Inexperienced students have a tremendous amount to learn. They have to take from the clinical data the kinds of things which clients say that show that they are anxious, or have changed the subject, or are beginning to distort something said yesterday, maybe for subconscious reasons. Verbatim notes do help the student to help the client. They provide enough accurate data to demonstrate the direction in which the nurse is going with the client. They also help the students to consider what the data tell them about themselves, to pick up recurring patterns of behaviour in the language of particular clients, and to consider what theories they need to help their clients. Peplau (1962) claimed that the learning product from verbatim recordings can be transferred at a later date to less formal contacts with clients.

One way of reducing some of the biases inherent in verbatim recording is to use some form of verbal classification system. Such a system provides a summary of the verbal interaction in an easily codified form; and can either be a popular coding schedule (e.g. Bales, 1950), specially useful for comparative research purposes, or one specially devised for specific teaching purposes (e.g. Marson, 1982).

Process Recording Following the Interview. This approach to process recording is a well established method of supervision with social work students in the United Kingdom, and some nurse educators in the United States use this method with basic students. At Highland College of Nursing one of my colleagues, who is a trained social worker, prefers this method and uses it with his students during clinical supervision. Students are required to record the content of their interactions immediately following the counselling interview with their clients. The students are instructed to record what they say and what the clients have said. They must also include their own feelings and inferences about the clients' feelings. Finally the students include a résumé of how the interaction has progressed. One advantage of this method is that the students are not distracted during the interview, and can concentrate entirely upon the verbal and non-verbal exchange as it occurs.

Some social workers have disputed that this form of process recording is accurate, claiming that many social work students fake the data. However, faking the data is less easy when supervisors interact closely with students and clients, as they should do here. A potential disadvantage with this method is that bias and distortion may occur even when the student is highly motivated. Advocates of the approach point out that with practice and experience, students can be trained to remember significant occurrences accurately and to omit subjective data. I accept that this is true, but only if the process recording occurs immediately after the clinical interview. Student nurses in the United Kingdom are not supernumerary members of the ward team, and may not always be able to record the interview immediately after it has occurred. The student's difficulties may be increased if the client talks rapidly, or if his/her verbal communication is bizarre.

Some teachers have attempted to minimise the problem of bias and distortion by reducing the duration of the interview to 10-15 minutes. My view is that this will sacrifice some of the potential gains from a thirty minute interview. The thirty minute interviews increase the student's opportunity to experience and overcome the problems encountered during relationship therapy. These problems occur at all phases of the relationship from orientation to termination, and include the personal feelings of the nurse and client. I believe that if a teacher reduces the interaction time, the student and client may attempt to reduce it further, until the contact time becomes insignificant. It is well established that many of the blocks in a helping relationship are blocks because both the nurse and the client use them as excuses to avoid each other.

Kagan has developed a form of process recall that reduces the possibility of bias — Interpersonal Process Recall (IPR) (see Kagan *et al.*, 1969; Kagan, 1973). In IPR trainees are asked to view themselves in interview with clients, on videotape, and to try to recall the feelings, thoughts, plans and actions that they experienced during the interview. IPR is widely used in both medical and nurse training in the USA and is gaining popularity in Australia; it has yet to be fully explored in this country.

Audiotape and Videotape Recording. Audio and videotapes are more accurate than handwritten methods of recording. They enable students to record all verbal communication, particularly when the client talks rapidly, and to record the nuances of the interview, which are of particular significance for psychiatric clients. They also allow the student to concentrate entirely upon the client's communication as it occurs. It is impossible to fake the data, even when the teacher's relationship with the client is superficial.

The disadvantage of both types of recordings is that they take longer to analyse than handwritten recordings; in other words, the volume of material is difficult to deal with. The amount of time required to analyse a tape recording is an important consideration, especially if the teacher intends to focus on psychiatric interactions other than clinical interviews, and intends to act as a role model for his/her students. Inexperienced students require a great deal of direction and interpretation, which tends to demand a great deal of the teacher's time. At Highland College of Nursing, teachers supervise up to five students at any one time in the clinical area, and it is for this reason that handwritten methods of recording have been preferred. Teachers in Inverness have elected to use audiotape recording with more experienced students to record and examine group interactions, during the progress of small therapeutic groups. In this situation, however, the teacher will not be fully involved with the ward milieu, and group therapy will be the main focus for the students' clinical teaching programme.

Videotape has obvious advantages in that it can include non-verbal as well as verbal behaviours, but with certain students (and clients) it can produce self-consciousness and anxiety: the playback must be handled sensitively and with care (Hung and Rosenthal, 1978). It is important to stress that teachers involved with clinical supervision must be very flexible. They must be prepared to compromise and use alternative methods when individual students present serious difficulties. The feelings and learning needs of the student must be placed before the teachers' personal biases. When teachers are supervising students during clinical interviews, they must take several factors into consideration. For example, they must consider the degree of student resistance or cooperation, problems in recording, the complexity of the teaching programme, and the experience and numbers of the students who are being supervised. Needless to say, decisions regarding informing clients fully of any method of recording will have to be made: there is rarely an excuse for not telling them.

In conclusion then, for the teaching/learning of counselling skills, some method of recording interviews with clients helps students to focus on their own and their clients' verbal behaviour, and to detect recurring patterns or habits in the speech; to perceive nuances in what clients say and strategies in what they, as helpers, say that may or may not be helpful; to develop the ability to collect some of the 'raw data' of therapeutic encounters, namely the verbal aspects; and to collect material for supervision sessions with their teachers that will form the basis of discussion regarding their personal and professional development, without requiring that teachers 'sit in' with them during their interviews. Methods of recording vary in their objectivity, but each has its attendant advantages and disadvantages, as discussed above. An additional reason for adopting some form of process recall is to encourage students to perceive the differences between empathy and sympathy.

Empathy and Sympathy in Therapeutic Relationships

Kalish (1973) emphasised that with empathy the helper remains separate and objective. By contrast, with sympathy, the helper experiences the clients' feelings as if they were her/his own. I believe that students can only understand the therapeutic significance of this difference if they experience both attitudes while being provided with close clinical supervision. Full understanding requires the ability on the part of the students to assess the impact of their attitudes and feelings upon the nurse-client relationship. A valuable aid to developing and monitoring self-awareness is the keeping of a daily journal or diary.

The Learner's Daily Journal

In order to help students to record their feelings and perceptions relating to their daily experiences and relationship with their teacher, the learner's daily journal is introduced to Inverness students during the first psychiatric nursing module, as an essential component of a client-centred teaching programme. The content is discussed each day at pre-clinical conference.

The purpose of this tool is to develop students' understanding of self, to identify milieu factors that facilitate or hinder students' learning, and to examine the student-teacher relationship. The insight gained into students' feelings and their perception of what was going on can be demonstrated by the following example of a student's comments:

> Immediately after this interaction (a shopping trip), the teacher asked me if it was beneficial. I said no: however, at the bus stop I felt awful for saying so, when in fact this was not true. I just felt tired and hungry, and I did not give his question any consideration. In fact I learned a lot about my client, as I had never seen her in that situation before.

If students are to make the most of their discussions with their teachers to encourage their own self-awareness, it is essential that a non-threatening relationship exists between them.

The Student-Teacher Relationship

In order to create such a non-threatening relationship, it is important to realise that the student-teacher relationship will progress through the same phases as the nurse-client relationship, namely (a) orientation, (b) testing out, (c) working together, and (d) termination. During the working phase of the relationship, students should feel free to express themselves, confident enough to interpret what is going on in their nurse-client relationships, and as a consequence grow in their ability to experiment with new ideas and skills. This description is very similar to Kalkman's (1967) description of the nurse-client relationship. I believe that the development of the student-teacher relationship is the most critical component of successful clinical supervision. If the relationship fails to develop beyond orientation or testing out phases, the teacher's ability to help students will be limited. A permissive, democratic supervisory structure will promote learning more effectively than an authoritarian structure in which the students are given directives and have less opportunity to reason through the problems for themselves.

In order to create such a learning environment, teachers themselves must be open and non-defensive, which will require a high degree of self-awareness. Their own nurse tutor training may not have adequately prepared them for this kind of teaching. If this is the case, it is essential that they, themselves, attend some training course(s). If teachers are defensive, it is likely that students will be unable to be open, and thus the opportunities for them to enhance their self-awareness will be reduced. Having created a non-threatening teaching relationship with students, teachers are then in a good position to provide role models for their students with regard to the core of the helping relationship. After all, teachers 'help' students just as nurses 'help' clients.

The Core of the Helping Relationship

Rogers (1965) identified three essential attitudes which he suggested were critical factors in the therapeutic relationship. These attitudes were described as genuineness in the relationship, a warm positive acceptance of the client, and an accurate empathic understanding of the client. Accepting that this is true, teachers in Inverness have attempted to impress upon their students during classroom teaching and clinical supervision that: (a) clients are responsible to varying degrees for their own actions; (b) accurate empathic statements facilitate the helping relationship; and (c) in order to be empathic we need to understand ourselves, and should continually evaluate our subjective attitudes and feelings.

In my view the daily review of journal content can contribute towards the development of the three essential attitudes identified by Rogers (1965) and can facilitate the student-teacher relationship.

Summary

Taking the teaching of counselling skills as an example, several themes have emerged that are pertinent to the learning, development and facilitation of IPS in psychiatric settings. Perhaps the most important issue to be identified is that those attitudinal and behavioural changes sought by teachers in their students will only occur when teachers demonstrate a willingness to practise what they teach. This will involve taking risks during interactions with clients and during clinical conferences with individual students. Teachers must develop their own levels of self-awareness and be ready to provide a non-threatening teaching context. This will enable students to increase the likelihood of their becoming more constructive in their (therapeutic) relationships with clients. The introduction of methods of process recall, and the discipline of keeping a daily journal, it was argued, are good ways of catalysing this awareness in students, and of helping them to identify their own strengths and weaknesses. In the context of counselling, it was argued that teachers should move out from behind their defensive cloaks of 'teachers', and that *all* nurse teachers should retain a dual classroom/clinical teaching role. The Inverness teaching programme could provide a model for this role in the United Kingdom.

Whilst this teaching programme has to some extent bridged the gap between theory and practice, we believe that a joint appointment, which allows teachers to take responsibility for nursing care prescriptions, is a logical future development. This development will ensure that theory bears a greater resemblance to practice particularly if it is combined with increased opportunities for research into psychiatric nursing, and a greater emphasis on the continuing education needs of trained clinical and teaching staff.

References

Altschul, A. (1972) *Patient-Nurse Interaction*, University of Edinburgh, Department of Nursing Studies. Monogram 3. Churchill Livingstone: Edinburgh

Bales, R.F. (1950) *Interaction Process Analysis*, Reading, Mass : Addison-Wesley

Boore, J. (1984) 'Nursing Research — Nursing Education' Janforum, *Journal of Advanced Nursing, 9*, 93-5

Caine, T. and Smail, D. (1968) 'Attitudes of Psychiatric Nurses to Their Role in Treatment', *British Journal of Medical Psychology, 41*, 193-7

Cormack, D. (1976) *Psychiatric Nursing Observed*, Royal College of Nursing Research Series, Royal College of Nursing: London

Ferguson, A. (1978) 'Psychiatric Nursing: The Myth Today', *Nursing Times, 74*, 1474-5

Hung, J.H.F. and Rosenthal, T.L. (1978) 'Therapeutic Videotaped Playback : a critical review', *Advances in Behaviour Research & Therapy, 1*, 103-35

Kagan, N. (1973) 'Influencing Human Interaction — Eleven Years of IPR', Paper presented at the *American Educational Research Association* Annual Convention: New Orleans

Kagan, N., Schauble, P., Resnikoff, A., Danish, S.J. and Krathwohl, D.R. (1969) 'Interpersonal Process Recall', *Journal of Nervous and Mental Disorders, 148*, 365-74

Kalkman, M.E. (1967) *Psychiatric Nursing*, McGraw Hill Company: New York

Kalish, B. (1973) 'What is Empathy?' *American Journal of Nursing, 73*, 1548-52

Marson, S.N. (1982) 'Ward Sister — teacher or facilitator?' *Journal Advanced Nursing*, 7, 347-57

Ministry of Health Report (1968) *Psychiatric Nursing Today and Tomorrow*, HMSO: London

Melia, K. (1981) 'Student Nurses' Construction of Nursing: A Discussion of a Qualitative Method', *Nursing Times*, 77, 697-9

Nicol, E. and Withington, D. (1981) 'Recorded Patient-Nurse-Interaction: An Advance in Psychiatric Nursing', *Nursing Times*, 77, 1351-2

Peplau, H. (1960) 'Talking with Patients', *American Journal of Nursing*, 60, 964-6

Peplau, H. (1962) 'Interpersonal Techniques : The Crux of Psychiatric Nursing', *American Journal of Nursing*, 62, 50-4

Reynolds, W. (1982) 'Patient Centred Teaching: A Future Role for the Psychiatric Nurse Teacher?', *Journal of Advanced Nursing*, 7, 469-75

Reynolds, W. and Cormack, D. (1982) 'Clinical Teaching: An Evaluation of a Problem Orientated Approach to Psychiatric Nursing Education', *Journal of Advanced Nursing*, 7, 231-7

Rogers, C. (1965) 'The Therapeutic Relationship : Recent Theory and Research', *Australian Journal of Psychology*, 17, 95-108

15 ISSUES ARISING FROM TEACHING INTERPERSONAL SKILLS IN POST-BASIC NURSE TRAINING

Carolyn Kagan

Introduction

There is a threefold need for some discussion of IPS in the context of post-basic nursing. Although there is growing recognition that some attention should be paid to the development of effective IPS in basic general and psychiatric nurse training (GNC, 1977, 1982), there is also recognition that trained nurses do not always use effective IPS in their work, at whatever level, and irrespective of nursing context (Ashworth, 1984; Faulkner and Maguire, 1984; Macleod Clark, 1983; Marson, 1982; Simpson, Back, Ingles, Kerckhoff and McKinney, 1979). *So there would seem to be a need for trained staff to receive some in-service education in IPS.* In Chapter 4, Ann Faulkner discusses some of the problems this poses with regard to availability of tutors, and management support or encouragement. There are many post-registration fields of nursing that require different and sometimes more specialised IPS (Briggs and Wright, 1982; Jones, 1983; McIntosh, 1981; Morgan, 1984; Westaby, 1983). Again, Ann Faulkner has discussed some of the issues with reference to community nursing in various forms (see Chapter 4). Ann Tait has described the special case of mastectomy nursing (Chapter 11). Despite the problems identified in these discussions, the various post-registration Boards require various degrees of consideration of IPS. *So there would appear to be a need for trained staff undergoing further professional training to receive some (more specialised) education in IPS.* In addition, I would like to suggest a further need for education in IPS. IPS are not skills that are learnt once and for all. Even if we were to reach a situation in nursing where all newly trained staff had had some IPS training, it would still be necessary for them to undergo refresher courses to review their own skills, and to develop them further. *So there is a need for continual review and updating of IPS in all fields of nursing.*

My own experience is primarily concerned with the second of these needs, namely IPS within the context of different post-registration

248

training courses, although I have had some involvement with trained nurses undertaking both in-service education with no prior experience of IPS, and personal/professional development either with/without prior IPS experience.

In this chapter, I propose to (a) present a model of IPS that I have found useful in designing IPS courses for different post-registration courses of various lengths; (b) discuss the needs of the different groups with respect to IPS; (c) outline some of the curricula that have been developed, and the ways they link in with other aspects of individual courses, and consider some of the problems of mounting and participating in the courses over the years; and (d) attempt an overall evaluation of IPS training course design and implementation with reference to individual and group needs of the students.

Before embarking on this enterprise, I must make some disclaimers (as, indeed, I must do each time I am faced with a new group of nurses!). I am not a nurse. I am a social psychologist with a special interest (and training) in the field of interpersonal relations. My research interests are related to problems that people experience in relating to and getting on with others (as experienced, for example by socially isolated or depressed people; professional people who meet difficult clients or who work in emotionally fraught situations; disadvantaged people such as people with mental handicap, women etc.). Since 1976 I have been involved in sharing these interests in a teaching capacity with a variety of vocationally dedicated students, as well as with undergraduates. Thus my 'expertise' with respect to nursing comes largely from what I have learned with my student groups over the years. I try to get a flavour of the different specialisms by spending a day or two with nurses in the field, and accompanying them as they go about their work. Perhaps most importantly, though, I have been a consumer of nursing services in paediatric, orthopaedic, acute medical, antenatal, delivery, post-natal and domiciliary settings. There is no doubt that all the students I teach know more about their work settings than I do, so it is essential that they get the opportunity to participate fully in the sessions.

To give the reader some idea of the scope of my teaching involvements, Table 15.1 presents an outline of the different nursing courses that I teach on, the numbers of students per class and the number of hours IPS work they have.

A Model of Interpersonal Skills

One of the major difficulties for IPS teaching is the lack of a simple model of IPS that not only incorporates some of the complexities of social interaction, but that is also able to incorporate both theoretical and practical issues. A further problem relates to the question of how to choose what to include in a course of a given length; there is no traditional syllabus content and an IPS course could fill as many hours as were allotted to it. There does not seem to be any 'natural' length for such a course: if experiential and practice sessions are included, an IPS course cannot be determined by the amount or sophistication of the theoretical material that could inform the subject. Given that post-registration courses are all of different lengths, and rarely include a *requirement* for an IPS component, a further constraint on curriculum design is imposed. (It is interesting to note that whilst the professional bodies do not *require* an IPS syllabus on most courses, they are generally pleased to see some coverage.) This raises a problem I shall return to later, namely the perceived status of IPS within a post-registration course.

I have found the following model useful in designing courses of different lengths, and for issuing to students so that they can see at a glance how those aspects of IPS they are covering in their course fit into a comprehensive model of IPS. Figure 15.1 is not a model of *how interpersonal relations occur.* It is, instead, a heuristic device that provides an overall conceptualisation of the *processes* involved in IPS. In addition to this model, I also use an adapted version of Argyle and Kendon's (1967) model of social skills as a useful means of conceptualising one-to-one interaction (see Chapter 2 by Davidson). Using Figure 15.1, and taking into account the needs of different groups of nurses as discussed in the next section, I use the 'topic and issue' areas represented in the circles, as the bases for the contents of individual syllabi. For each circle, or 'module', there is a discrete theoretical background, set of practical skills and relevant and appropriate assessment that can be identified. Whichever 'module' is under consideration, the influence of the environmental and social context, including social/cultural rules, roles and rituals, must also be taken into account.

The figure is not supposed to imply that at all times each 'module' is equally important. It is, more appropriately, that the 'modules' assume differential importance for different groups and/or individuals at different times. The advantages of this model are that:

Table 15.1: Interpersonal Skills Teaching on Various Post-basic Training Courses at Manchester Polytechnic

Course	Student Numbers and Experience	Length of IPS Course	Assessment Required
Community Psychiatric Nursing (ENB 810)	c. 30 p.a. Some with prior knowledge of the community	c. 15 hrs as part of 27 hour 'academic' social psychology course. More included in sessions relating to professional nursing practice, elsewhere on course.	One piece of written work contributing to final result.
Community Mental Handicap Nursing (ENB 805)	c. 15 p.a. Some with prior knowledge of the community		
Certificate in Occupational Health Nursing: Day Release (RCN)	c. 25 p.a. All working in occupational settings	4 sessions, as part of 14 session Psychology course (a few 'Counselling' sessions included elsewhere)	None
Certificate in Occupational Health Nursing: Full Time (RCN)	c. 20 p.a. Most with prior experience in occupational settings		
B.Sc. Nursing Studies (CNAA)	c. 15 p.a. Varied clinical experience	73 hrs IPS in Nursing course (some communication and developmental/social psychology included elsewhere)	Two pieces of written work to contribute to final result. One 3-hour Finals examination.
District Nurse Certificate RGN (ENB)	c. 25 p.a. Some with prior experience in the community	5 sessions of 16 session psychology course (under review) (More included by DN Tutors)	One piece written work (not usually in IPS)
District Nurse Certificate SEN (ENB)	c.20 p.a. Some with prior experience in the community	Under review	
District Nurse Practical Work Teachers Course (ENB)	c. 17 p.a. All experienced and qualified DNs	1 session + whole day as part of 2-day Counselling course (More included by DN Tutors)	None
Health Visitor Fieldwork Teachers Certificate (ENB)	c. 20 p.a. All experienced and qualified HVs	Whole day as part of 2-day Counselling course (more included by HV Tutors)	None
District Nurse Supervisors of Supervised Practice Course (ENB)	c. 25 p.a. All experienced and qualified DNs (mostly NOs)	Half a day (more included by DN Tutors)	None

Figure 15.1: A Model of Interpersonal Skill

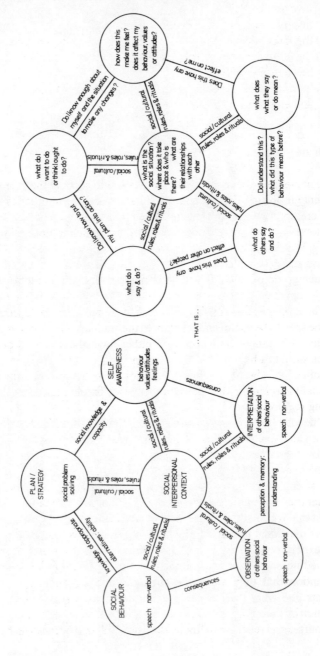

(1) it provides an overall view of many of the complex processes involved in IPS;
(2) discrete 'content' areas can be identified;
(3) the links between discrete 'content' areas can be easily seen;
(4) the influence of the environmental/social context can be seen to be central (sic); and
(5) 'performance' aspects of IPS are put into the context of cognitive and emotional aspects.

Needs of Different Student Groups

I have mentioned above the necessity to take into account the 'needs' of different groups in planning courses. *I* have to do this in order to have some credibility with my students, given that I am not a nurse. There are, however, two more important reasons for taking note of them. Firstly, IPS do not take place in a vacuum: they are to some extent constrained and determined by the nursing context (see Chapters 4, 5 and 6.) Each group of students will be bringing with them a unique set of nursing contexts, and if the classes are to bear some relevance, cognisance must be taken of them. Secondly, in the field of IPS, courses must be seen to be useful and relevant to the students if common myths, such as 'IPS cannot be learnt, you either have them or you don't'; 'nurses wouldn't be nurses if they weren't good at IPS' etc. are to be combatted. This latter point becomes particularly important if the professional validating bodies put IPS low down on their list of essential training requirements.

By 'needs', I refer to the *perceived needs* that the students themselves have, and not needs as defined by professional 'experts'. By saying this I do not mean to imply that all nursing students are so fully self-aware that they can perceive their own professional requirements and personal strengths and weaknesses with regard to IPS, regardless of whether they have previously considered IPS or not. Instead, I want to suggest that if IPS sessions are to be of any value at all to the students, trainers must take into account what these students already know and have experienced. It is, in my view, quite arrogant for any trainers, qualified nurses or not, to approach post-basic IPS courses with the assumption that they *know* the strengths and weaknesses of their students and what their working environment is/was like. Full participation by the students will ensure the most effective use of time on an IPS course, and teaching methods to ensure that this occurs will be the most valuable.

I would like to summarise some of the perceptions that different groups of students of mine have held, with regard to their 'needs' from an IPS course. At the start of any course, I ask students 'What problems with communication or interpersonal skills do you experience in your work?' A summary of replies given by students during the past few years is presented in Table 15.2. Whenever possible, I try to incorporate these issues into the teaching. Students are asked to keep a copy of their 'personal needs' for reconsideration at the end of the course.

Having obtained some idea of student group requirements, and taking into account any recommendations for syllabus content offered by the professional bodies, I design courses in consultation with the specialist nursing staff. It is essential, though, that the courses remain flexible enough to incorporate particular student interests and preferences that emerge during the course, if the course is to be meaningful to the students.

Course Curricula

In this section, I hope to show how the model of IPS (Figure 15.1) is used for the design of different curricula, and how these are implemented with regard to teaching methods and assessment (for a full discussion of curriculum design in nurse education, see Greaves, 1984). I have chosen three courses with which to illustrate the process. The courses differ with respect to the length of the IPS component and its links with other aspects of the course; student interest; topics covered and problems encountered.

Community Psychiatric and Mental Handicap Nursing

The content of the course for Community Psychiatric and Mental Handicap Nurses, with reference to the model of IPS is shown in Figure 15.2.

As Table 15.1 shows, the IPS course is part of a more general Social Psychology course, one requisite of which is that students must demonstrate a conceptual grasp of theoretical issues. Thus the course cannot focus exclusively on 'performance' aspects of IPS. The classes are large (approximately 45 students), and CPN and CMHN students are taught as one group. Each session lasts for three hours, including a break.

The sessions consist of a large experiential component, a shorter 'lecture' component (about 30 min.) and small group discussions of central themes emerging from the exercises and lecture. Handouts relating to the theoretical issues, with fairly detailed reference lists, are provided. Any of the sessions could be used as the basis for the written assessment. The topics included for each 'module' are summarised in Table 15.3.

Figure 15.2: Course Content: Community Psychiatric and Community Mental Handicap Nursing

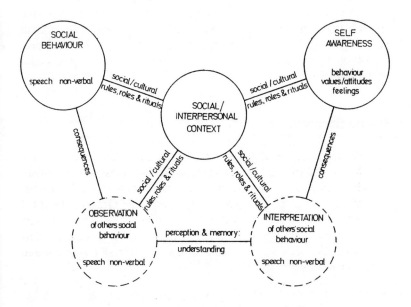

Throughout the course, attention is paid to the therapeutic value of some of the skills and issues. In other words, not only do students consider their *own* IPS, but also how they can extend their knowledge and awareness into therapeutic sessions with clients. Thus, Social Skills Training sessions are also included for use with psychologically disturbed clients, mentally handicapped people and junior staff in training of, for example, counselling and other helping skills. The assessment is two-pronged: students choose one from a number of topics, covering the whole course. For each one, they are asked for a theoreti-

Table 15.2: Problems of Communication/Interpersonal Skills Experienced in Different Work Settings

Problems identified by more than 20% respondents	CPN N=129	CMHN N=30	OHN N=125	DN N=52	HV N=30	DNPWT HVFWT N=42	Hospital[a] N=25
Personal Constraints							
How to handle emotionality in others	*					*	*
Arrogance	*	*					
Inability to listen at times	*	*			*	*	*
Lack awareness other carers' roles	*	*		*	*		
Reluctance to share information	*			*	*		
Intolerance of others' views	*					*	
Role conflict		*					*
Reluctance to communicate with relatives	*	*		*	*	*	*
Lack experience with particular clients				*	*		*
Ambiguous communications					*		*
Rigid values				*	*	*	*
What to say to dying people and their relatives	*						*
Inability to convey precise information briefly	*						*
Embarrassment at touching							*
Like/dislike some patients more than others				*		*	*
Avoid difficult questioning				*			*
Poor timing of giving information	*						*
Avoid speaking to unconscious patients	*			*			*
Organisational or Professional Constraints							
Lack of coordination between departments	*	*	*				*
Too few telephone lines	*	*	*		*		*
Other professionals unavailable	*	*			*		
Management does not pass necessary information	*			*			
Poor information on discharge from hospital	*			*		*	
Lack of knowledge about nurse role by others	*	*	*			*	

Poor communication with medical personnel

Difficulty of access to information

Decisions made about clients by others without consultation

Shift work

Management insensitive to demands and gives little support

Lack of privacy

Poor organisational facilities

Senior staff seem threatened

Supercilious attitudes of medical staff

Routine

Need to attend to machines

Language difficulties (Senior medical staff)

Rigid Management structure

Client Constraints

Nature illness/handicap

Lack confidence in nurse

Language difficulties

Lack motivation (to change)

Misperception nurses' role

Overdependence

Rigid attitudes

Domestic circumstances

Overconfidence

Inability to assimilate information

Inability to assimilate unfavourable news

Degrees of sensory deprivation

Children do not understand

Isolation

[a] including nurses working in midwifery; intensive care/therapy units; general medical, geriatric, surgical paediatric, orthopaedic wards; infection control; clinical teaching settings.

Table 15.3: Content of IPS Sessions: CPN/CMHN

Session	Experiential	Theoretical
Social Context	Variability of own behaviour according to situation, role and other people	Person-Situation debate
(2 sessions)	Self Concept	Self Concept
	Institutional design and the control of behaviour	Physical, social and ritual aspects of environments and the effect on interaction
Social behaviour	Description own nvb Changing nvb	Description and functions nvb
Non-verbal behaviour	Nv expression emotion Nv expression interpersonal attitudes	Cultural and subcultural variability in nvb Expression *v.* interpretation
(1 session)		
Language (1 session)	Explanation and information Latent *v.* manifest meaning Defences and blocks	Social functions language Language rituals Codes and Meanings
Self-Awareness	Values, attitudes & beliefs Prejudice (+/−) Sexual Identity	Nature and function values, attitudes and beliefs Prejudice and person perception
(2 sessions)	Attribution sexuality Role Conflict	Sex roles, role and role conflict Self awareness and consciousness
Observation and Interpretation	incorporated in all of the above sessions	

cal discussion based on the literature, and then in some way to show that they can apply this knowledge practically. In the context of IPS, this may be, for example, to devise a staff training programme in specified helping skills; to design living accommodation for clients with specified interaction difficulties; or to identify the source of some enduring characteristics they, themselves, possess, and so on.

The Social Psychology course takes place in the first of three terms and runs in parallel to Psychology and Sociology courses. Links with these courses are drawn throughout lecture and discussion components. Furthermore, later in the course, other tutors dealing with issues of professional practice pursue IPS work in detail, often with the aid of videotaped playback. Thus the Social Psychology course provides an introduction to many IPS issues and concepts that are examined in detail elsewhere on the professional course.

Problems Encountered in Teaching the CPN/CMHN Course. It is difficult teaching CPN and CMHN students together. The contexts in which they work are generally very different, and they experience diverse barriers to the effective use of IPS. However, the problems are only really significant for the lecture component: here it is my responsibility to ensure that the content is relevant to both sets of students. During the experiential sessions students bring their own examples and discuss pertinent applications: thus, here it is the responsibility of the students themselves to ensure relevance. Mixed CPN/CMHN discussion groups are useful, too, for widening the scope of the discussion to the mutual benefit of all. It can sometimes be difficult structuring the exercises meaningfully for both groups: however, student comments have helped me modify the exercises over the years, sometimes leading me to drop some completely, but at other times simply helping me introduce them differently.

With this course, there is little opportunity for me to pay individual attention to students, and I am not in a position to evaluate individual skills. I can comment on the practical component of the assignment, but this is not the same as commenting on people's *performance*. However, as indicated above, the professional nursing practice sessions do afford students the opportunity to examine their own IPS in detail.

Some of the students have had quite extensive backgrounds in psychological/social psychological theory and often experience of different therapies. It can be difficult, therefore, pitching the lecture input at the appropriate level. Generally, though, the students are highly motivated and interested in the practical applications of the issues, and do not disrupt the sessions, even if they think 'they've heard it all before'. One last thing that is striking, is that it is crucial that enough time is left at the end of each session for individual students to 'work through' issues that have personal relevance for them. Feelings and reactions are often evoked that surprise and sometimes disturb students: not only must I be prepared to give time to students who have such experiences, I must also be prepared (and able) to handle emotional distress. This is common to all experiential teaching of IPS, and such reactions do not always confine themselves to the end of sessions. At times, emotional reactions must be handled in the class situation. I would strongly advise any tutors who feel unable to handle conflict, fear, anger etc. in the classroom, to try to attend some training sessions in experiential teaching/learning techniques before they attempt to use them.

Certificate in Occupational Health Nursing Course

The content of the course for Occupational Health Nurses, with reference to the model of IPS is shown in Figure 15.3. As indicated in Table 15.1, the IPS sessions are part of a general 'Psychology' course which includes a large amount of organisational/occupational psychology. Students are always keen to discuss issues that are broadly to do with 'dealing with people', 'stress' and 'group decision making'. The Psychology section is part of a heavily prescribed course that contains a great deal of work to be assessed and passed for the award of the Certificate. There is no assessment requirement for Psychology. The classes are fairly large (20-25 students), most of whom are generally women. Each session is 2½ hours long, including a break. The sessions are primarily experiential. Handouts containing theoretical material and references relating to the exercises and topics are provided. Students usually process their reactions to the exercises in the whole group, rather than in small groups (this is not always so large — see 'Problems' section below). The topics included for each of the IPS sessions are shown in Table 15.4. Throughout the processing, students are encouraged to relate the exercises to their particular work contexts, which they do readily. Some of the issues raised are followed up in other Psychology sessions, and occasionally in Sociology sessions, but otherwise there is little opportunity to develop themes or pay attention to issues that arise for individual students elsewhere in the course. A very small 'counselling' course is included that affords the opportunity to develop some of the 'performance' issues that are raised. On the whole, though, the course is so heavily prescribed with other subjects that are crucial for the award of the Certificate that very little importance is placed on IPS work.

Problems Encountered in Teaching the OHN Course. I have experienced more difficulties with these courses than with any other course in my teaching career. The difficulties are related to the structure of the Certificate course and the importance placed on IPS work, student attitude and motivation, and my own inability to meet the needs of the students.

The course is, as I have said, a full one, requiring extensive coverage of many subjects with compulsory assessments. Students are therefore always inundated with course work and assignments that must be of a

Figure 15.3: Course Content: Occupational Health Nursing

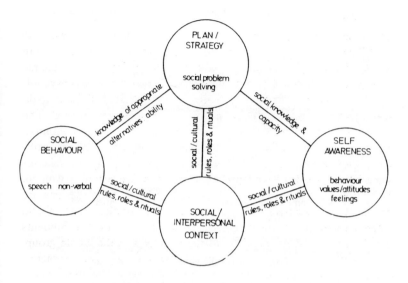

satisfactory standard if they are to be awarded the Certificate. Thus, they have 'better things to do with their time' than attend Psychology classes that are not essential to the course and they stop attending Psychology classes. It is unfortunate that students are 'forced' to be so instrumental in their approach to the course, but until the RCN acknowledges the importance of IPS work in the training of Occupational Health Nurses, the situation is understandable, and will I am sure continue. In this context then, students find IPS a waste of time. Many students, however, do experience conflict over this, as they feel that a large part of their work as an OHN is concerned with relating to people in counselling, conflict and often welfare situations. Furthermore, they frequently feel inadequately prepared to 'help' clients who are depressed, anxious, angry, upset, suffering from occupational or personal stress, experiencing marital and/or sexual discord, and so on.

And yet there is another dimension of student attitude that combines with this perceived need to look at IPS on the course. I have found that OHN students are more rigid than any other group of students I teach. This rigidity is manifest in two ways. Very many times I have been told that 'we don't need to discuss this — we wouldn't be nurses if we weren't good at relating to people', or 'the moment I decided to become a nurse

Table 15.4: Content of IPS Sessions: OHN

Session	Experiential	Theoretical
Social Behaviour Non-verbal behaviour (1 session)	Description own nvb Communication emotion Communication interpersonal attitudes Conveying complex messages on noisy factory floor Establishing rapport Observation of groups and individuals	Description and function nvb Expression *v.* Interpretation Environmental conditions and their effects on nvb
Language (1 session)	Latent and manifest meaning Blocks and defences Communication status Recording language	Social functions of language Latent *v.* manifest meanings Language rituals and codes
Self-Awareness (1 session)	Life events, stress and depression Social manipulation and need for approval Variability behaviour according to role, situation and other people Public *v.* Private selves	Individual differences and person-situation debate Social motivation Susceptibility to stress Nature of depression Self presentation
Social Problem Solving (1 session)	Role-played small-group decision making (a) allocating overtime (b) allocating redundancies	Small group dynamics

was the moment I realised I was good at getting on with people', and so on. These views stick, even in the face of contrary 'evidence' during exercises ('the exercise was silly . . . '). The other way that rigidity reveals itself is in the students' reluctance to engage in any experiential learning: they want the *facts* — the information — about IPS and related issues. These 'facts' are difficult for me to provide, as I believe very strongly in the variability of individual IPS with the situation, and the importance of the influence of the environmental/social context. Because of my preference for experiential teaching/learning, and my reluctance to look at IPS as if there were facts to be learnt about them, I may not be the best person to teach OHN students, given that many of them have a preference for didactic teaching/learning methods. Indeed, I no longer teach these courses. I have, though, included discussion of

I no longer teach these courses. I have, though, included discussion of them here in order to illustrate two points.

It is difficult, but sometimes necessary, to acknowledge that in the area of IPS teaching, a particular tutor may not be able to meet the needs of a particular group of students; this is particularly difficult for the tutor her/himself to acknowledge. I am lucky in that I work in an organisation that is large enough for me to be able to exchange some courses with a colleague. Where there is no alternative but for the tutor to continue with the groups of students, some compromises might have to be made with regard to both course content and teaching methods; this may mean that the original goals for the IPS course may not be fully met, which can be unsatisfactory for everyone concerned. The second point I wish to emphasise is that student motivation and professional recognition are inextricably linked. Lack of professional recognition of the role of IPS in a training course can occur in any field, and student motivation is likely to suffer as a result.

Figure 15.4: Course Content: B.Sc. Nursing Studies

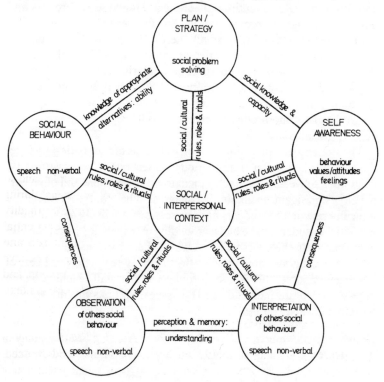

BSc Nursing Studies Course

The content of the course for the BSc Nursing Studies students, with reference to the model of IPS, is shown in Figure 15.4.

As Table 15.1 shows, the IPS course is a long and comprehensive course that continues throughout the third and fourth years of the four-year degree course. Two pieces of assessed work are required in the third year, and the course culminates in a three-hour unseen finals examination paper. Students are expected to demonstrate conceptual grasp of theoretical issues but, as I shall discuss later, they are also required to demonstrate some practical ability. The classes are small (between 7 and 15 students) and are taught as one group. Students come from a variety of clinical fields including midwifery, community, health visiting, psychiatry, community psychiatry and mental handicap, paediatrics, geriatric, general surgical and medical, basic and post-basic education, occupational health, theatre and intensive care. The length of each session varies according to the content of the course (see Table 15.5). The course runs over five terms: the first two are experiential, the third a mixture of experiential and theoretical, and the fourth and fifth terms almost entirely theoretical. Handouts, references and directed readings are provided in the last two terms.

Because the classes are so small, there are opportunities for discussion of issues that are of particular interest to individual students throughout the course. It is possible, particularly in the second term, to pay individual attention to a variety of IPS, both at the micro-level of examining specific verbal or non-verbal elements, or at the more macro-level of interpreting roles and developing strategies/plans to achieve social goals.

The students are all working as nurses and, as the course is part-time, they are able in the intervening period to reflect on the issues we discuss from week to week: this enables them to bring pertinent and often personally significant examples to classes. The course is therefore topically relevant to students and the sessions are lively and stimulating. All the students have had a grounding in 'psychology over the lifespan' earlier in the course and so, whilst their previous knowledge of psychological issues may vary, by the time they reach the third year of the degree course, this is not a problem. Other staff teaching on the degree course are interested in IPS issues, so links are drawn continually between courses.

Problems Encountered in Teaching the B. Sc Nursing Studies Course.
The degree course is primarily an academic course and initially

students find the experiential emphasis of the IPS component disconcerting. However, they do very quickly appreciate the relevance of the
course to their work as it proceeds, and thus they participate with great
enthusiasm. The enormous diversity of experience among students can

Table 15.5: Content of IPS Sessions: B.Sc. Nursing Studies

TERM 1: fortnightly sessions of 3 hours

Session	Experiential	Theoretical
Models of Interaction (1 session)	Identification of the elements and components of interaction	Models of interaction, communication and social skills
Social context (1 session)	Variability of own behaviour according to situation, role and other people Self and personality Situational boundaries	Person-situation debate Perception and meaning of situations
Social behaviour		
Non-verbal behaviour (2 sessions)	Describing own nvb Nv expression emotion Nv expression interpersonal attitudes Nvb in patient care: case studies	Description and functions of nvb Cultural and subcultural variability in nvb Expression *v.* interpretation Nv communication in patient care
Language (3 sessions)	Information and explanation Giving bad news Conversation analyses: simple-complex Links between nvb and language	Language and the regulation social behaviour Social functions Language rituals (in nursing contexts) Codes and meanings

Assignment

(1) Collect a sample of speech between two people and critically comment
on it; *or*
(2) Observe (a) a person alone; (b) 2 people together in time and space; (c)
2 people interacting; (d) a group of people interacting; (e) a group of
people interacting of whom you are one. Indicate what you
observed, what this meant, and how you felt as observer.

TERM 2: fortnightly sessions of 3 hours

Series of videotaped role-plays with feedback. Emphasis on own verbal and non-verbal behaviour, and on analysing the tapes with reference to the effects of behaviour on others; distinction between observation and interpretation; possibilities of behaviour change; public and private self-awareness and self-consciousness; strategies of coping with role conflict and personal confusion. Analysis of pre-recorded nursing interactions, with emphasis on the social meaning of speech and non-verbal behaviour, and the situational/personal/organisational constraints on social behaviour. Social goals and social problem solving.

TERM 3: weekly sessions of 1 hour

Student seminars. Students to take turns in (a) presenting an academic paper on IPS in specific nursing contexts; and (b) organising and chairing the sessions.

Peer evaluation of (a) presentation of the paper, including use of visual aids, handouts etc. and content; and (b) the skills of organising and chairing the sessions.

Discussion of small group dynamics

Assignment

Theoretical discussion of choice of topics concerned with IPS in nursing.

TERM 4: weekly sessions of 1 hour

Theoretical discussions relating experiential work in Terms 1-3 to research findings in social psychological and nursing investigations. Handouts and references provided.

TERM 5: *c.* 5 hourly sessions prior to examinations

Integration of experiential and theoretical work, serving as revision sessions. Discussions based on case studies brought by students

Exercises (again for revision purposes) concerned with the critical appraisal of research in IPS in nursing.

ASSESSMENT

3 hour unseen Finals paper. 3 questions to be answered from 8, covering most of the IPS syllabus. One of these is compulsory and is designed to tap the practical skill of conversation analysis. Students are presented with a conversation between a nurse and another person (usually a patient), and are asked to comment on it critically, incorporating any knowledge about IPS they wish to. Some examples of the conversations are given at the end of the chapter.

sometimes be difficult to handle, especially towards the beginning of the IPS course, as so much of the discussion is related to personal experience. However, after a few sessions, students know a great deal about each other's work settings and can constructively comment on the issues that are raised.

The experiential work in the second and third terms with its emphasis on performance, can be traumatic, and students sometimes experience considerable discomfort. With this course, though, we are lucky in that student numbers are small, the course is long and the sessions can be unhurried. Thus there is ample time for the whole class to deal with each other's worries and frustrations in a positive and constructive way. Not only does this alleviate the particular person's discomfort, but the other students begin to acquire ways of handling personal distress, and of making constructive criticism. There is rarely time to explore these themes in an IPS component of a professional training course, and the students profess to find the experience useful at work. Interestingly, the discomfort experienced by students is generally greater during the third term, when they are having to 'perform' both interpersonally and academically.

The last problem I have in working with the B.Sc. group is of how to devise a realistic set of assessments that do not subordinate practical skills to academic debate. I think we have reached a fair compromise, tapping a wide range of skills, but the assessments are continually under review. Unfortunately it is about the only issue on which students have few, if any, helpful coments to make regarding change. For details of the assessments see Table 15.5.

District Nursing and Health Visiting Courses

I will not go into details about these courses here. I will, however, give a summary of the course content, with reference to the model of IPS presented in Figure 15.1, to indicate the focus of each course. They all have their attendant problems, but in some form or another these have all been covered in the discussion of the three courses above.

Figure 15.5: Course Content: District Nursing

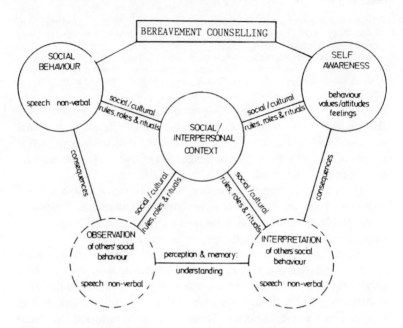

Evaluation of IPS Courses in Post-basic Education

Ann Faulkner (Chapter 16) has considered the evaluation of teaching IPS in some detail, and I do not intend to anticipate here much of what she will say.

On the post-basic courses on which I teach there are different requirements made by the validating bodies regarding assessment. None of the professional bodies asks for evaluation of *IPS per se* (whether this be performance, observation, interpretation, self-awareness or social problem-solving skill). Where some assessment is called for, I have tried to balance theoretical knowledge with the ability to apply this knowledge in meaningful ways (see discussion of CPN/ CMHN and B.Sc. Nursing Studies courses above). I do not think that 'testing' students on their knowledge of the research findings in the field of IPS in nursing is any test of practical ability at all; nor do I think that assessment of practical ability should be confined to *performance*. All the 'modules' of Figure 15.1 are potentially of importance, and in some contexts some will assume greater importance than others. They are all potentially 'assessable'.

Figure 15.6: Course Content: District Nurse Practical Work
Teaching and Health Visitor Fieldwork Teaching

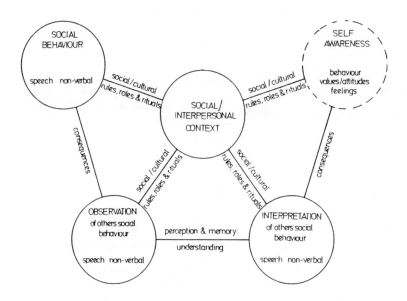

A further problem of assessing IPS is that they are not 'once and for all' skills that students have either learnt or they have not. IPS are flexible and continually changing according to the nature and demands of the situation. The demonstration of a certain level of skill in one situation at a particular time is no guarantee of skill in different situations or at different times. Perhaps we should be trying to tap this flexibility of skill in assessment, that is, attempting to assess the process of using IPS rather than the end product of the employment of a particular skill or set of skills. Indeed, there is contemporary discussion, in the clinical and social psychological fields, of the possibility that those who are most socially skilled and better adjusted are those that are the most flexible and responsive to changing circumstances, and that can perceive the nuances of different social situations. That is, they are the most 'socially intelligent'. (See D'Zurilla and Nezu (1982) and Kagan (1984) for some discussion of this.)

Certainly, there is rarely only one *right* way of interacting: the skill is largely in perceiving the need to change the style of interaction and of being able to effect this change. Ultimately, the assessment linked to an IPS (as with any) course must be related to the educational objectives of

Figure 15.7: Course Content: District Nurse Supervisors of Supervised Practice

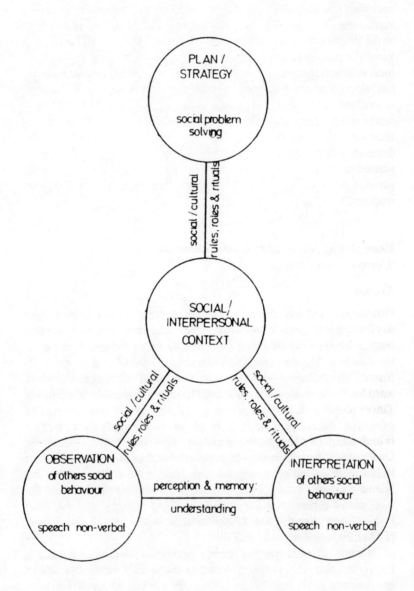

the course, and in order to construct meaningful assessments it may first be necessary to construct meaningful courses! In addition, for those students for whom there is no formal assessment requirement, it will be necessary, in assessing the value of the course, to *ask the students* themselves. That is, to see whether the needs identified by the students at the beginning of the course have been met. Only the students will know the answer to this, so we must ask them. Their answers can be most telling, but we must trust them enough to know whether the course has 'worked' or not. Providing they are given sufficient time at the start to explore their own needs, I believe they can and will assess themselves and the course meaningfully. If we are to involve students fully in the course, though, the tutor-student relationship is an important one to develop in a constructive way, and Bill Reynolds (Chapter 14) has considered this in some detail. If we want nurses to be open and honest with patients, then we, as tutors, must be open and honest with our students.

Examples of (shortened) Conversation for 'Conversation Analysis'

Example 1

Patient (P): Woman (48 years). In hospital for D & C. Arrived yesterday for D & C to be performed today. Four children 18-25 years. Never been in hospital before except to have first two children.

Nurse (N): 2nd year student nurse. Been working a busy Gynaecology ward for seven weeks. Is popular and a good student (according to both Tutors and Ward Staff).

Ward: Busy 16 bed Gynaecology ward attached to two consultants. Understaffed and relies on students to provide minimal nursing care.

P Nurse!

N Just a minute, love. I'll be with you in a tick. (After a few seconds, approaches foot of P's bed)

P You know, I'm not sure what all this is about.

N Oh now, don't you worry. You'll be all right. It'll be over before you know it, and . . .

P . . . Yes, but what exactly are they going to do? I don't really know what a . . .

N Oh yes you do. It's just a little procedure that lots of women your age have. It's nothing to worry about. Now, you're not going to worry about it any more, are you?

P But D & C — what does it mean?

N Everybody knows about it — you just ask any of the others — they'll tell you.

P Nurse — *what* does D & C stand for?

N It stands for . . . oh! — I don't know!

Example 2

Patient (P): Elderly woman (78 years). Recently returned from hospital where she had an artificial hip put in. Lives with sister (73 years). Nurse visits daily to assist with washing, as she is still a bit unsteady on her feet.

Nurse (N): Community Nurse (30 years) new to the area. Has been visiting patient every day since she returned from hospital 1½ weeks ago. Just come back from long weekend off. It is 8.00 a.m. as she enters patient's bedroom.

N Hello Elsie love, it's me again. How are you? Time to get up? Not in bed still?

P Who's me? Oh, you. I'm having a lie-in, nothing to get up for.

N Now then. How did you get on with Sister Walker? Nice isn't she? Come on now.

P Ouch.

N Swing your legs over, that's right.

P Did you get them, then? Like you promised?

N Yes I did. But I'm not going to give them to you until you're up. Hold on now. Ooo, gosh, you weigh a ton.

P Less of your cheek.

N Less of your own. Now, where is it? Ah, here. Do your teeth then.

P All right, all right, don't nag.

References

Argyle, M. and Kendon, A. (1967) 'The Experimental Analysis of Social Performance' in L. Berkowitz (ed.) *Advances in Experimental Social Psychology*, *3*, 55-98, Academic Press: New York

Ashworth, P.N. (1984) 'Staff-Patient Communication in Coronary Care Units', *Journal of Advanced Nursing*, *9*, 35-42

Briggs, K. and Wright, B. (1982) 'A Fundamental Skill', *Nursing Mirror*, September, 34-6

D'Zurilla, T.J. and Nezu, A. (1982) 'Social Problem Solving in Adults' in P.C. Kendall (ed.), *Advances in Cognitive Behavioral Research and Therapy, 1*, Academic Press: London

General Nursing Council for England and Wales (1977) *Training Syllabus for Register of Nurses* GNC: London

General Nursing Council for England and Wales (1982) *Training Syllabus for Register of Nurses: Mental Nursing* GNC: London

Greaves, F. (1984) *Nurse Education and the Curriculum: a curricular model*, Croom Helm: London

Faulkner, A. and Maguire, P. (1984) 'Teaching Assessment Skills' in A. Faulkner (ed.) *Recent Advances in Nursing, 7 Communication*, Churchill Livingstone: Edinburgh

Jones, P. (1983) 'Teaching Communication' *Nursing Times, Community Outlook*, 10 August, 229-30

Kagan, C. (1984) 'Social Problem Solving and Social Skills Training', *British Journal of Clinical Psychology, 23*, 161-73

Marson, S.N. (1982) 'Ward Sister — Teacher or Facilitator? An investigation into the behavioural characteristics of effective ward teachers', *Journal of Advanced Nursing, 7*, 347-57

McIntosh, J. (1981) 'Communicating with Patients in their Own Homes' in W. Bridge and J. Macleod Clark (eds), *Communication in Nursing Care* HM & M: London

Macleod Clark, J. (1983) 'Nurse-Patient Communication: an analysis of conversations from surgical wards' in J. Wilson-Barnett (ed.) *Nursing Research, Ten Studies in Patient Care*, Wiley: Chichester

Morgan, A. (1984) 'Learning to Interact', *Journal of District Nursing*, April, 20,22,24

Simpson, I.H., Back, K., Ingles, T., Kerckhoff, A. and McKinney, J.C. (1979) *From Student to Nurse: A longitudinal study of socialization*, Cambridge University Press; Cambridge

Westaby, J.R. (1983) 'Communication and the Occupational Health Nurse', *Occupational Health Nursing*, December, 22-5

16 THE EVALUATION OF TEACHING INTERPERSONAL SKILLS TO NURSES

Ann Faulkner

Introduction

The traditional way to evaluate if teaching has been successful is by written examination and, in nursing, by assessment of practice on the ward. Because the statutory bodies controlling nursing have the function of protecting the public, emphasis has been on whether or not the nurse is a safe practitioner. Evaluation to measure if the teaching of interpersonal skills has been effective presents many problems, not least in deciding what exactly is to be measured. Zusman and Bissonette (1973) suggest that 'evaluation, like any potentially potent tool, can do more harm when used clumsily than if not used at all'. If, for example, interpersonal skills were to be measured by written examination there might yet be a discrepancy between what is written and what happens in patient care (Bendall, 1975). If ward-based interpersonal skills were assessed, difficulties could arise in what in fact the examiners interpreted as interpersonal skills.

Such problems of interpretation do not arise in other areas of nursing. In physical care there are clear expectations of what nurses should be able to do at different points in their training. Skills in terms of giving injections, making beds or giving bedbaths, for example, are clearly defined. There is no such clear definition of interpersonal skills. In Faulkner, Bridge and Macleod Clark's (1983) survey of directors of nurse education, there was not even agreement on how much time would be spent teaching the subject, nor at what point it should be taught, during training.

A further dilemma in evaluating the teaching of interpersonal skills arises from the possibility that little or no *formal* teaching may have been given on the subject, and there are ethical issues in evaluating aspects of care which may not have been taught to the learners. In order to develop evaluation tools to measure interpersonal skills, decisions need to be made on which skills nurses are expected to develop at particular points in a training programme so that appropriate methods of measurement may be used. Thus the evaluation of teaching interpersonal skills is no different from assessing the teaching of any other skills, in so far as it must follow from the learning objectives, curricula content and teaching methods. Evaluation *per se* is meaningless.

The Need for Baseline Data

In order to know if teaching has been effective, it is necessary to have some baseline data from the learners. One could argue that there is a large research literature to suggest that nurses do not possess interpersonal skills (e.g. Ashworth, 1980; Faulkner, 1980; Macleod Clark, 1982; Maguire, Tait and Brook. 1980). However, although such research findings highlight the problems in nursing, they do not give a tutor any idea of how well an individual nurse can perform without tuition. It is reasonable to expect that entrants to nursing will start their training with a wide variation in interpersonal skills, ranging from the shy learners who need to develop confidence to the extroverts who may need to subdue some of their natural 'bounce' in certain situations. Baseline data on how learners might interact with a patient will not only alert a tutor to the needs of the group but will also allow individual progress to be measured.

There are a number of ways of collecting baseline data. Faulkner and Maguire (1984) asked nurses to make an audio-tape of an interview with a patient, using a structured assessment form as a guide for areas to be covered. This study was concerned primarily with the development of assessment skills but the method could be extended to other areas where interpersonal skills are important, such as patient education, counselling and more general social interaction. These initial audio-tapes were used not only to teach nurses but to measure any improvement in skills after training by comparing first and later recordings.

Faulkner (1980) used vignettes of patient situations to ask nurses how they would react in certain situations. A similar approach is being used in one of the written tests currently being developed by the Communication in Nurse Education (CINE) Project, which is funded by the Health Education Council (HEC). Other written tests are also being developed and tested within the project, to give some indication of nurses' abilities at the start of training in the area of interpersonal skills. These tests are interesting in that they do not attempt to measure *behaviour*. Rather they are concerned with some of the cognitive aspects of interpersonal skill, in this case problem-solving and planning.

Yet another method of collecting baseline data is by videotaping interactions. There are some difficulties here in terms both of bulky apparatus and the strain new learners may feel if they are expected to interact with a patient and be filmed *before* they have had any formal tuition. In the CINE project, baseline data of this type are being collected by filming role-play sessions between learners, where one takes the part of nurse and the other takes the part of patient. The problems inherent in role-play are discussed by Anne Tomlinson in Chapter 12 of this book. Here it is enough to say that role-play situations appear to give a reasonable indication of current interpersonal skills in preset situations, although the extent to which the skills generalise to other situations is questionable.

If baseline data are not collected, any future evaluation of learners will be measuring an individual's performance rather than the effect of any teaching on the subject. Further, it will be impossible to take account of individual differences in skills before teaching had occurred. One could argue that the important point *is* eventual performance of the nurse, but if interpersonal skills become an accepted, important part of curricula, it is necessary to evaluate the teaching of those skills, and this may best be done by measuring *differences* in nurses' performance before and after teaching of the necessary skills. In assessing the durability of any teaching of interpersonal skills it will be necessary to conduct 'follow-up' studies over a period of time, especially as the contexts in which the skills are to be displayed may vary considerably. Attempts to assess changes in social behaviour over time are fraught with methodological problems. Some helpful suggestions on planning such investigations are given by Cook and Campbell (1979).

In measuring change over a period of time, in order to evaluate the teaching of interpersonal skills, it has to be accepted that in real life situations there are many variables which cannot be controlled, not least the expectations of ward staff where nurses gain their practical experience. These variables may affect the nurses' perceptions of what they have been taught and so influence their priorities. The effect of uncontrolled variables may mean that any differences measured in interpersonal skills may not be attributable to the teaching programme alone. Zusman and Bissonette (1973) state, 'When we are dealing with human services and human problems the number of possible causative variables is staggering.' This must be as true in nursing as in any area where human behaviour is being monitored.

What *is* known from available research is that qualified nurses do not generally exhibit effective interpersonal skills on the ward, so it may be tentatively suggested that any differences in the performance of learners undergoing training are likely to be due primarily to teaching. If in-service education programmes in interpersonal skills are developed for trained staff, it may be more difficult to differentiate learning formally in the school from learning informally on the wards.

Post-teaching Data

If evaluation of teaching is designed to measure differences in performance from baseline to post-teaching tests, there would appear to be a strong argument that baseline and post-test material should be identical. In Faulkner and Maguire's (1984) study, ward nurses' baseline and post-test audiotapes were both of the assessment of a mastectomy patient after operation, using a standard assessment form. The patients were different, which could be seen as an important variable, but it was argued that the skills of assessment would not vary, although cognisance was taken of the fact that an articulate patient *could* (and probably would) affect outcomes. This effect has been shown by Fairbairn, Maguire, Chambers and Sanson-Fisher (1983) where an experienced teacher appeared to perform little better than a novice, apparently because patients interviewed by their students spontaneously volunteered more relevant information than patients of other teachers in the study on baseline interviews.

In current work of Faulkner and Maguire, the assessment skills of community nurses have been measured before and after brief training. Difficulties have been found, in that baseline audiotapes have been on *first* post-discharge assessment of mastectomy patients, while post-test audiotapes have been of *follow-up* visits to the same patient. An unexpected variable which may have affected results here is that the community nurses in the study do not appear to see the need to re-assess their patients after the initial visit. This illustrates the problems of evaluation in a real life situation.

If baseline and post-teaching evaluation depends on the same material, it could be argued that learners will do better simply because of a practice effect. Given that there will be a reasonable time lag between baseline and post-tests, it is unlikely that learners will remember what they have written. Not only that, if nothing has been learned, then there are unlikely to be differences in responses. If, however, the initial assessment had been used for feedback and teaching purposes, there is a distinct possibility that this would distort the post-teaching data.

Factors to be Measured

Whichever method is chosen to collect evidence of nurses' ability to interact with their patients and colleagues, the task which besets the teacher or researcher is how to analyse the material to give a clear picture of whether skills taught have been learned.

Young (1982), in discussing the need to measure nursing skills, illustrates with a section of an evaluation form headed 'understanding patients' needs'. This form deals with the areas of 'understanding' and 'responding', and 'carrying out', but does not appear to attempt to measure the nurses' interpersonal skills in assessing the patients' needs. If teaching is to be evaluated so that teachers can make necessary adjustments to their material, evaluation will need to be precise.

Some aspects of interpersonal skills, notably verbal skills, can be readily identified, such as the ability to ask questions. It can be seen if nurses use open and closed questions appropriately, if they use brief single questions rather than long multiple questions and if they ask leading questions. Other areas such as the use of jargon, blocking, missing cues and making assumptions without clarification may also be observed for their presence or absence. Notes may be made on the nature of greetings and closures of interactions and of the nurses' willingness to allow patients to disclose their concerns.

Those ill-defined areas such as empathy and warmth are more difficult to evaluate, since here judgements have to be made about nurses' feelings when they react to an individual. This is also a difficult area to teach. Davis (1982), for example, found that nurses after empathy training were likely to give more stereotyped reassurance than those nurses who did not receive training. Evaluating empathy has to be more than looking at words or gestures used for if, for example, a patient describes some trauma in her/his life, the response 'poor you' could be empathetic, bored, sarcastic or simply mechanical. This illustrates rather nicely the need to consider the *interaction context* of interpersonal skills and to avoid focusing on what just *one* person (i.e. the nurse) in the context does or says.

In written tests, some notion of what is expected in an answer should be identified. This can cause difficulties if the material is 'open' as in Faulkner's (1980) vignettes, since some means of categorising or analysing the content of the vignettes will need to be developed. Having an 'ideal' answer may be less useful than identifying strategies which teachers could expect nurses to use after teaching them the relevant interpersonal skills.

Methods of Measurement

Analysing interpersonal skills has been of concern in both education and the social sciences for a considerable time, but Diers and Leonard (1966), in discussing interaction analysis, suggest that 'methods used must be relevant for the practice of nursing', and go on to suggest a need to adapt social science methods to the study of nurse-patient interaction.

If nurses' interpersonal skills are to be measured from recorded material, audio or audio-visual, a choice may be made between making decisions direct or from transcripts. Much will depend on what is to be extracted from the data. If, for example, utterances are to be counted and categorised, it can be argued that transcripts might be easier to deal with. However, a transcript is devoid of all but the words of an interaction and as such may not measure if teachers have met their objectives in terms of what students have learned. Macleod Clark (1982), in analysing nurse-patient interactions, found difficulty in reaching agreement with others in analysing transcripts of nurses interacting on a surgical ward. She also found difficulty if raters were shown videotaped recordings of the interactions, and concluded that the rating systems may not have suited the data to be analysed. This work illustrates some of the problems in evaluating interpersonal skills teaching especially if it is seen in very general terms. The task becomes easier if teaching concentrates on areas of interpersonal skills that are needed by all nurses, or identifies specific skills that are to be developed.

In the nursing process approach to care (McFarlane and Castledine, 1982), it can be seen that every nurse needs the skills of assessment, the skills to impart knowledge and the skills of counselling (although not all would agree on the point in training at which such skills are required). If interpersonal skills are subdivided in this way, methods of evaluation will look for specific behaviour which can, hopefully, be measured.

In measuring nurses' performance, scales are often used which measure general behaviour on scales from 1 to 4 (e.g. Young, 1982). Young uses a general behaviour (among others) of 'responding to patients' requests for attention'. Nurses can score as follows:

1 Sometimes lacks perception
2 Alert to patients' needs most of time
3 Meets patients' needs quickly and competently
4 Poor response to patients' needs

Young describes this as an improvement on gradings which go from best to worst, but it is still using a normative approach which in effect compares nurses against each other and an 'ideal' behaviour. Furthermore, raters have to make the choice between alternatives: thus the measure may be one of raters' perceptional skills rather than nurses' expressive skills! Krumme (1975) makes the case for criterion referenced measurement which 'judges an individual's performance against specific behavioural criteria'. She criticises normative reference methods on the grounds of subjectivity, and describes a situation where a scale was used without prior definition of what constituted 'superior', 'above average', 'average', 'below average' and 'unacceptable'. This meant that evaluators were left to make their own interpretation and judgement. This is very different from criteria referenced judgements where nurses are judged 'purely on whether or not they have met the performance criteria'.

Criteria referenced measurement would seem appropriate for judging nurses' ability to interact with their patients. Faulkner and Maguire (1984), in evaluating the teachers of assessment skills, used a modified form of a scale described by Maguire *et al.* (1978) for measuring medical students' ability to interview. Although it can be argued that a medical interview may be different from a nursing assessment, the techniques may be seen to be common.

The techniques as described by Maguire *et al.* (1978) were as follows:

Clarification
Avoiding jargon
Rejecting jargon
Handling of emotionally loaded material
Controlling the interview
Avoiding repetition
Picking up verbal leads
Encouraging precision
Facilitating
Use of open questions
Use of brief questions

Faulkner and Maguire (1984) rated nurses on a 0-4 scale for each of the techniques where 0 equalled total omission and 4 equalled very good use of the technique with no omissions. Each nurse gained a total score on both baseline and post-teaching audiotapes so that observations could be made on the level of improvement. Overall ratings were given on self-assurance, empathy, warmth and competence, although these had not been taught. It can in fact be argued that if nurses learn the elements of interviewing, they will become competent. Competence brings self-assurance, and empathy may develop as nurses learn to understand their patients. If this is so it could be argued that 'empathy training' could be both unnecessary and unproductive. However, this is a theoretical debate and requires further empirical support to substantiate the argument one way or another.

Similar criteria could be developed to measure other aspects of interpersonal skills. The value of this approach to evaluation is that distinct areas may be isolated where improvement is needed, and encouragement may be given to learners when they meet some of the criteria. From current research, for example, nurses are found to be very effective in controlling assessment interviews and in avoiding repetition, but very poor in questioning techniques, and in handling emotionally loaded material.

Inter-rater Reliability

If methods of evaluation are to be meaningful, then the criteria against which a nurse's performance is measured must be interpreted in the same way by each evaluator, that is, they must be reliable. Methods must also be validated. Macleod Clark (1982) improved inter-rater reliability from 30 per cent (poor), to 70 per cent (acceptable) after she had devised an analysis procedure specifically designed to categorise her communication material. This reflected an attempt to make the categorisation system relevant to the data and not a distortion of the data to make them acceptable.

In the medical field, interaction analysis has long been seen as an effective method of evaluating the teaching of interviewing skills. Scott, Donnelly, Gallagher and Hess (1973) suggest that evaluation of students has 'tended to be loose, unstructured and highly subjective . . . ', and make the case for direct interaction analysis, reporting high levels of inter-rater reliability. Maguire *et al.* (1978) also report high levels of inter-rater reliability when evaluating the teaching of interviewing skills to medical students, using a specific categorisation system. Faulkner and Maguire (1984), too, showed very high levels of inter-rater reliability when evaluating nurses' assessment performance. Each criterion was clearly defined in a manual, and precise instructions were given of possible responses and of how they would be scored.

It is usually suggested that raters need training. Scott *et al.* (1973) thought that the use of untrained raters would lower inter-rater reliability. In Faulkner and Maguire's current research, one rater was highly trained and the other completely untrained but experienced in teaching interpersonal skills. Inter-rater reliability was very high, suggesting that if criteria are clearly defined and the rater is experienced in the subject to be evaluated, then training may not be necessary.

If tutors wish to evaluate interpersonal skills by analysing interactions, then at least two raters should be used. Total agreement on overall scores cannot be expected since individual differences affect perception, but agreement should be high (and the higher the better) if the criteria for assessment are reliable and valid.

Work in this area suggests that evaluation of interpersonal skills does not require transcribing before analysis. Transcription only serves to reduce the amount of information available for analysis: it does not allow tone, pitch, speed of voice and hesitations, for example, to be taken into account. This is important if tools are to be developed to evaluate a nurse's performance in the clinical setting, and if the skills to be evaluated are the total range of interpersonal behaviours, rather than simply the verbal content.

Interpersonal Skills in the Clinical Setting

The aim of teaching interpersonal skills is that nurse will acquire skills and give priority to meaningful interaction with patients and staff in the clinical setting. This suggests that even if nurses are evaluated in the classroom there remains considerable value in evaluating their performance with patients.

Egert (1975) describes a *'challenge exam'* to evaluate students' performance with clients. This examination allowed the student to choose a classmate, friend or client to counsel and also allowed collaboration between nurse and client before the event. However, it was found that the exercise was fear-provoking for the students even though they had explanatory guidelines prior to videotaping of the counselling situation. Furthermore, it could be described in terms of role-play rather than a real life situation, and is, therefore, subject to the criticisms outlined above. Scoring, to see if nurses had met the 'challenge', was by two tutors who averaged their scores. Another method which could possibly be developed to evaluate a nurse's performance in the clinical field is that of patient satisfaction. This is an area which has received little or no attention except by researchers. At a personal level it has certainly been found that patients are tremendously loyal to nurses while they are patients. Any minor criticisms are usually followed by comments on how hard the nurses work and how much is expected of them. Possibly patients feel a fear of retribution if they complain, since certainly the major complaints from ex-patients remain in the field of communication. If patient satisfaction were to be used as a method of evaluating interpersonal skills in the clinical setting, assurances of confidentiality would need to be given, and patients would need to understand that their constructive comments would help nurses to develop their skills. Problems arising might be in the area of bias and subjectivity, as this method assumes a certain degree of perceptiveness on the part of the patients. It would be difficult to match such an evaluation with teaching objectives, unless these, too, were couched in terms of aiming to increase patient satisfaction. Other areas of clinical practice are evaluated on the wards. If appropriate tools were developed, there seems little reason why interpersonal skills should not also be evaluated as a nurse interacts with a patient in the clinical setting, although few of these other skills are assessed by the patients themselves!

One method for evaluation of interpersonal skills could be similar to that used by Faulkner and Maguire (1984). Nurses could tape-record a prescribed interaction with a patient and complete a written account of their interaction. Tutors could then evaluate skills by coding the audiotape and written account according to predetermined criteria. A second assessor could be used so that reliability of evaluation could be assured. An advantage of this method would be that nurses could record their interactions when they felt ready to do so, without the stress of an observer's presence.

An immediate disadvantage is similar to that described by Egert (1975), in that, by allowing a nurse to choose, evaluated interactions may only be those with pleasant articulate patients. However, it can be argued that if nurses are skilful with cooperative patients, they have learned the required skills and, hopefully, would be able to use them with less amenable patients; the counter-argument is that different skills are necessary for interacting with the different patients. Another disadvantage is that of time. If two tutors have to rate interactions separately, the exercise becomes very time consuming. Further, an extensive supply of tape-recorders would be required so that when particular students were ready to record their interaction, equipment was readily available.

In current research with trained nurses the idea is emerging that a nurse's interactions could be coded on the ward by two assessors. The requirements are clearly defined criteria and a rating scale for each criterion which is readily understood. It has been shown that Maguire *et al.*'s (1978) scale can be used by an untrained rater. This scale certainly lends itself to development in areas other than assessment. Those tutors evaluating interpersonal skills would need to be experienced in the teaching of those skills, for although Fairbairn *et al.* (1983) suggest that this work can be carried out by inexperienced teachers, the numbers used in the study were small and may not be representative. Certainly, in the CINE study, tutors who have not had preparation in teaching interpersonal skills feel very vulnerable and are often loath to take on such teaching.

A disadvantage of direct evaluation on the ward is the effect observation may have on the student. This is already a problem in evaluating clinical skills, and time and thought need to be given to methods of reducing a learner's anxiety and any effects this may have on performance. There may also be a question of patient cooperation, and perhaps it is presumptuous to assume that patients will automatically agree to cooperate. In current research with trained nurses patients have been very willing to cooperate in order to help the nurse to develop such skills, and it is already usual for patients to take part in a nurse's assessment of drug rounds, for example. As long as patients are given a clear option, it seems unlikely that it would be harmful to them to evaluate a nurse's competence in a real life situation.

Obviously much work needs to be carried out before ideal tools exist to evaluate the teaching of interpersonal skills. Hopefully, current research will provide some of the answers.

Conclusions

This chapter has discussed evaluation of teaching interpersonal skills. Possibilities have been seen to exist to measure improvement from baseline data by using written material, which will show if underlying concepts have been understood. In order to show if skills have been learned however, it has been suggested that evaluation of audio-visual, or actual interactions should take place. At the present state of knowledge, evaluation of such material would need to be on criterion rather than normative measures, with criteria clearly defined so that the method was reliable between raters. If actual interactions are to be evaluated in the clinical setting, observer effects would need to be minimal to reduce learners' anxiety.

The priority remaining, however, is the appropriate and skilful teaching of interpersonal skills. Until this becomes an integral part of all curricula for nurses, and until tutors themselves possess the skills to teach using experiential methods, evaluation will remain vague and clumsy, and mostly a glib written exercise. Nurses will continue to write 'would reassure the patient' while examiners will continue to wonder 'what about?'

Acknowledgements

I would like to acknowledge the other CINE directors, without whom the project would not exist — Will Bridge, Jill Macleod Clark and Jane Randell. Also, Brian Neeson who is research officer (evaluation), and the HEC for funding. An acknowledgement is also due to Peter Maguire, with whom I am collaborating on the work with trained nurses, for his help and confidence in the work, which is funded by the DHSS.

References

Ashworth, P. (1980) *Care to Communicate*, RCN: London
Bendall, E. (1975) *So You Passed, Nurse?* RCN : London
Cook, T.D. and Campbell, D.T. (1979) *Quasi-experimentation: Design and analysis issues for field settings*, Rand McNally: Chicago
Davis, B.D. (1982) 'Social Skills Training', *Nursing Times*, *78*, 1765-8
Diers, D. and Leonard, R. (1966) 'Interaction Analysis in Nursing Research', *Nursing Research*, *15*, 225-8
Egert, L. (1975) 'Challenge Exam in Interpersonal Skills', *Nursing Outlook*, *23*, 707-10
Fairbairn, S., Maguire, P., Chambers, H. and Sanson-Fisher, R. (1983) 'The Teaching of Interviewing Skills: comparison of experienced and novice trainers', *Medical Education*, *17* 296-9
Faulkner, A. (1980) 'The Student Nurses' Role in Giving Information to Patients', unpublished M Litt thesis: Aberdeen University
Faulkner, A., Bridge, W. and Macleod Clark, J. (1983) 'Teaching Communication in Schools of Nursing: A survey of Directors of Nurse Education', Paper given at RCN Conference: Brighton
Faulkner, A. and Maguire, P. (1984) 'Teaching Assessment Skills 'in A. Faulkner (ed.), *Recent Advances in Nursing*, *7*, *Communication*, Churchill Livingstone: Edinburgh
Krumme, L.L. (1975) 'The Case for Criterion-referenced Measurement', *Nursing Outlook*, *23*, 764-70
Maguire, P., Roe, P., Goldberg, D., Jones, S., Hyde, C. and O'Dowd, T. (1978) 'The Value of Feedback in Teaching Interviewing Skills to Medical Students', *Psychological Medicine*, *8*, 695-704
Maguire, P., Tait, A. and Brook, M. (1980) 'A Conspiracy of Pretence', *Nursing Mirror*, *150*, 17-19

Macleod Clark, J. (1982) 'Nurse-patient Verbal Interaction', *unpublished PhD thesis* University of London

McFarlane, J. and Castledine, G. (1982) *A Guide to the Practice of Nursing*, Mosby: London

Scott, N., Donnelly, M.B., Gallagher, R. and Hess, J. (1973) 'Interaction Analysis as a Method for Assessing Skill in Relating to Patients: Studies on validity', *British Journal of Medical Education*, 7, 174-8

Young, A.P. (1982) 'Measurement of Nursing Skills — the search for a suitable assessment tool', *Nursing Times*, 78, Occasional paper

Zusman, J. and Bissonette, R. (1973) 'The Case Against Evaluation', *International Journal of Mental Health*, 2, 111-25

POSTSCRIPT

Carolyn Kagan

Introduction

This final chapter gives me the opportunity to comment on some of the
aspects of interpersonal skills in nursing that have received fleeting
attention elsewhere in the book. It provides me with the chance to
clarify what I consider to be crucial concerns for both research into, and
applications of, interpersonal skills in nursing. In a sense, the very
choice of chapters and writers, and the way I have structured the book
reveals my orientation. What I intend to do here is to highlight issues
that will be discussed for some time to come.

A skills approach to interpersonal behaviour is one that celebrates
the individual. The individual learns, or is taught, appropriate skills,
and is then expected to put them to good use. When research shows that
nurses do not put appropriate interpersonal skills to good use, the
asumption tends to be that they lack those skills. As we have seen,
though, it is possible to identify many factors that might inhibit or prevent individual nurses from using those skills they possess and, indeed,
do put to good use in non-nursing situations. It seems to me that this
issue is central to the whole field of interpersonal skills in nursing, and
can be expressed in the form of a question:

If we discover that nurses use ineffective interpersonal skills, are we
justified in suggesting that this is due to lack of skill rather than to
constraints on the use of the skills?

The Scope of Interpersonal Skills Research and Application

Most of the research and applications of interpersonal skills in nursing
that have been discussed in this book have focused on *performance*
components of skill (both verbal and non-verbal), usually in the form of
conversations between nurses and patients. There is a danger that the
performance picture has been distorted, as analysis of segments of an
interaction out of context, or the analysis of entire interactions in the

287

absence of information about the relationships between the people involved and knowledge about their understanding of the situation they are in, can be misleading. This emphasis also portrays a narrow view of the nature of interpersonal skill, as it excludes the examination of other features of interpersonal skill as well as other types of interaction.

There has been little discussion of cognitive aspects of interpersonal skill, and in many ways I think these are more crucial than the performance aspects. By cognitive aspects, I mean those that relate to the knowledge and understanding of which behaviours are appropriate in a particular situation, given certain interaction goals. Included in this is the appreciation of social and socio-linguistic rules underlying different situations (both explicit — i.e. clearly stated — and implicit — i.e. assumed through cultural and/or subcultural tradition), and the recognition and acknowledgement of one's own and other people's attitudes and values. Furthermore, the knowledge of alternative strategies that may be used to achieve interaction goals is necessary. These cognitive components combine to social problem-solving ability, and if interpersonal skills are considered at this level, I suggest that a more flexible and responsive use of performance skill will result. Nurses will be able to respond to unexpected behaviour from their interaction partners, whether they be patients, relatives or colleagues. They will also be able to 'save' an interpersonal situation that had not been going according to plan: they will be able to deal with the outcomes of both good and poor displays of interpersonal skill. We should, then be asking:

What role do cognitive components of interpersonal skill play in effective interpersonal performance?

Throughout the book, the emphasis has been on one-to-one interactions, generally between nurses and patients. Nursing does, however, include many different types of relationships in different interaction settings. Team meetings, ward reports and case conferences all require group interaction skills. They all, too, involve interactions with colleagues who may differ in terms of role, status and interpersonal skill. In these situations, an understanding of role within the particular health care organisation may be called for, and this will involve exploration of values, attitudes, prejudices, likes and dislikes. Frequently, too, nurses may be required to employ assertion skills. It is interesting to note that assertion has barely been discussed in this volume, and yet this set of skills is fundamental to a great deal of nurses' work. Assertion can include the eliciting of information, persuasion, negotiation, accepting positive appraisal and self disclosure as well as the ability to manage the conversation (begin and end it, and keep it 'on task' if necessary). It is not only with colleagues that nurses need to use group, and often assertion, skills. Take for example, the skills that the black ward sister will need in order to defuse overt racial conflict between patients: or those that the health visitor will need when she finds herself caught up in the conflicts between members of a family as they introduce an elderly relative to their household. We need to know:

How does the work on interpersonal skills in nursing help nurses deal with group situations they are faced with?

The Definition of Appropriate Interpersonal Skill

This leads me to reflect on who it is that decides which interpersonal skills are the important ones. This is a central concern for research, as it underlies the choice of subject matter to be studied. It is also central to the teaching of interpersonal skills, as it underlies both the content and assessment of courses. I suggest that both researchers and teachers should ensure that the skills they have chosen to focus on are the ones that nurses, patients, and anyone else involved consider to be the most meaningful and helpful to them. It is not enough for researchers and teachers to plan their projects with reference to previous research and theory, as this might mean they would be repeating the 'mistakes' that had been made.

To a certain extent the research questions, methods and designs will dictate the findings that emerge. The construction of interview questions and other research tools is complex, and requires that a great deal of time is spent on their form and structure. Many a research investigation includes leading or even closed questions in the name of experimental design. Even 'loose' methods that encourage free expression frequently determine what is to be included or excluded. In order to make sense of research findings, and to assess their value for future investigations, it is usually necessary to examine the research tools. This is, however, rarely done, and the next piece of research takes as its starting point the findings alone. As research progresses, we should ask:

How, exactly, was the previous research carried out?

Most of the writers in this book offer the same solution to those inter-personal skill problems revealed through the research — training. The expectant optimism with which training is offered leads us to believe that once nurses have learnt or been sensitised to the 'correct' interpersonal skills, they will use them effectively and the quality of patient care will improve. However, there are, I think, several inherent difficulties in this line of thought. In many ways, specialist interpersonal skills are easier to identify for both research and training, and it may well be that the success of teaching will lie mainly in these areas. Even then, though, the decision as to what level of skill is acceptable must be made. Are we talking about *good* interpersonal skills, or *good enough* interpersonal skills, and how do we distinguish between them? If interpersonal skills do become central to the assessment of good nursing practice, will nurses be excluded from the profession if they are not good enough? If so, who will set the criteria and be the judge of individual nurses? (If not, why not?) Will good *overall* skills be distinguished from good *specialist* skills, and which will be preferred? Will nurses who are only good with child patients be prohibited from nursing adults? We can summarise these questions by asking:

How will interpersonal skills be assessed in the overall judgement of acceptable nursing practice? How will these assessments be used with reference to the professional development of individual nurses?

The Place of Emotion in Interpersonal Skill

The place of emotional arousal — frustration, anger, upset, humiliation, elation and so on — in the use of interpersonal skills has been given little attention, and yet this, too, is crucial, especially in an emotionally charged occupation such as nursing. Unless nurses are encouraged to acknowledge their emotional involvement in their work and to believe that such reactions are normal, and are given the opportunity to express their feelings with the necessary professional support, their relationships with patients and colleagues may be distorted. Instead of relationships built on the honesty and openness they hope to engender in patients, nurses will relate to others from behind facades constructed to protect themselves from emotional hurt. We must address the question:

What is the place of emotion in the effective use of interpersonal skills by nurses, and how can appropriate support systems be ensured?

It is not only in practical nursing that the role of emotion should be considered. We have seen that interpersonal skills teaching requires special relationships between teachers and learners to develop. The tutor-student relationship will have to be founded on non-defensiveness, openness and honesty, and this in turn means that nurse tutors will have to acquire new, and often threatening teaching skills. Without this genuineness, attempts to teach interpersonal skills to nurses will fall short of their possibilities. It is, therefore imperative that we consider the question:

How can the essential requirements of genuine tutor-student relationships be encouraged?

Teaching Interpersonal Skills

The quality of tutor-student relationships will emerge as the teaching of interpersonal skills grows. For both the teaching and implementation of interpersonal skills to be successful, we have seen that cooperation between all those (potentially) involved is ideal. Not only that, but it is possible. If it does prove difficult in any particular situation, we should perhaps consider including in our teaching the interpersonal skills that are required to gain cooperation and maintain goodwill. The skills of working cooperatively are rarely considered in discussions of interpersonal skills in nursing, and yet so much nursing activity requires them to be used. It is unhelpful for nurses to employ 'all' their interpersonal skills effectively when relating to patients, but then to go on to be curt and dismissive to colleagues. Patients can be made to feel very uncomfortable if they overhear such encounters, and staff morale may well be affected (with its attendant consequences for patients). It would be worth spending some time considering:

What are the skills of cooperation between health workers, and how can they best be taught to nurses?

There is another reason for clarifying the nature of interpersonal skills, especially for the teaching/learning of those skills. If skills are not learned thoroughly or are used incompetently, they may result in increased patient distress. Several of the authors in this volume have alluded to the possibility that partially 'correct' skills may be more damaging than no skills. Two examples of this immediately spring to mind. I was recently talking with an Oncology group about counselling dying and bereaved people. On the issue of 'to tell or not to tell' patients about the nature of their diseases, I was faced with the protest ' . . . but when we tell them, quite clearly, they go away and we then find out, much later, that they'd got completely the wrong end of the stick . . . ' So the information had been given, but the health workers *failed* to check patients' understanding ('It was clear to me, so it must have been to them . . . '). Similarly, I witnessed a reasonable attempt to prepare a patient for a series of investigations into the paralysis of her left arm. The X-ray procedure was painstakingly explained to her: she was told she would have some coloured liquid injected into her backbone to colour the nerves, so they would show up on the film; they could then see if anything was wrong with them; . . . and so on. Simple, clear information, so why did the patient become extremely distressed? Because for her 'nerves' meant madness. Again, the explanation had been given, but understanding had not been checked. It was assumed she would know what nerves were. Following teaching we will need to know:

> How often are interpersonal skills mislearnt or misapplied?
> What effect does this have on patient well being?

This last example also illustrates a further problem in identifying appropriate interpersonal skills for teaching. That is, the role of subcultural variations in the use of language and non-verbal behaviours. Language style can vary enormously from region to region in Britain, and the use of euphemism prevails — perhaps more in the health field than anywhere. Parts of the body, bodily processes and so on are talked about differently in different subcultures. Can the middle class Londoner relate closely to the working class Mancunian; or the white nurse establish rapport with the Rastafarian youth or Asian primigravida; or the patient from the Potteries understand the humour of the Glaswegian student nurse? Given the complexities of informal social relations, there may be a case to be made for nurses acquiring a more formal speech style that transcends cultural/subcultural boundaries. If they were to do this, they would lose the advantages of establishing informal relationships with patients, which might be more important. The question remains though:

What notice will be taken of subcultural knowledge and skill in the assessment and teaching of interpersonal skills?

Future Prospects

My final comments relate back to the issue of individual responsibility for the effective use of interpersonal skills. The National Health Service is undergoing yet another reorganisation with the introduction of 'general management'. Nurses, along with other health workers, are in a position of uncertainty about many aspects of their work and the organisational structures of which they are a part. This uncertainty is bound to affect their use of interpersonal skill in ways hitherto uncharted. At some point nurses may feel that patient well-being is subordinated to organisational convenience to such an extent that they must take a stand. It will be interesting, then, to see if the nursing establishment that supports many of the current developments in interpersonal skills research, training and application, will extend its support to facilitating the protest, negotiation and patient advocacy skills that will be essential if the quality of patient care is to be maintained.

The questions to be asked of interpersonal skills in nursing will, then, probably be political, and the applications almost certainly will be.

INDEX